Renal Diet

COOKBOOK
FOR BEGINNERS

Let's Talk Diet! Preserve your Kidney Health with these 300 Easy Make Recipes - Low Sodium, Low Potassium, and Low Phosphorus Renal Diet Recipes

Kat Wildman

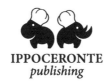

IPPOCERONTE
publishing

CONTENT

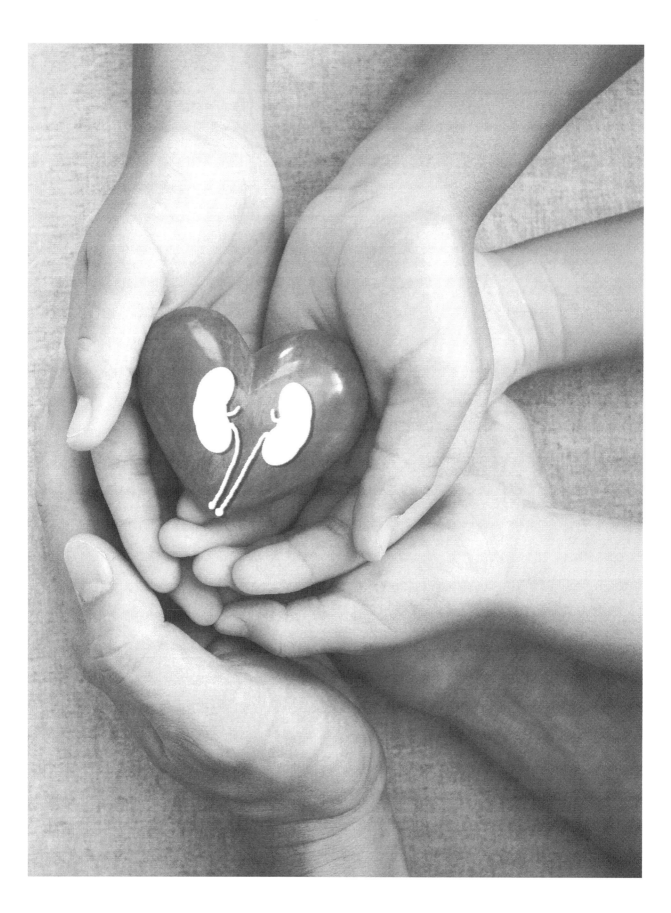

Introduction

Taking care of your daily diet is important because it plays a crucial role in your overall health and well-being. What you eat affects pretty much all the major organs and systems present within your body. This becomes even more important if you are dealing with any challenge associated with the functioning of a major organ. In such instances, the first thing you must do is ensure that the diet you consume does not worsen the situation and, instead, promotes internal homeostasis and better organ health.

One of the most important organs responsible for maintaining your overall health is the kidneys. Kidneys are your body's waste filtration system. They not only remove waste, but excess fluid present within as well. They are responsible for the excretion and reabsorption of all the essential chemicals and nutrients your body needs to ensure it is functioning effectively and efficiently. Any health condition or disorder that harms kidney functioning can have a significant effect on your overall health as well.

Living with a kidney disease is not easy and it can be downright challenging on certain days. A few lifestyle and dietary factors can worsen this condition. Whether it is diabetes, obesity, or an unhealthy diet, different lifestyle factors can increase the stress on the kidneys. The good news is, with a little conscious effort and consistency, you can ensure that this does not get in the way of living your life. If you want to regain control of your life and improve the health of your kidneys, you should try the renal diet.

The renal diet, as the name suggests, is a healthy eating pattern for promoting the health and functioning of the kidneys. Different complications are associated with kidney problems such as imbalance of electrolytes and anemia. In such instances, several micronutrients, such as phosphorus, potassium, sodium, and fluid input, are restricted. When significant dietary changes need to be made, having the necessary and proper information is needed. This is where the concept of the renal diet steps into the picture. Apart from ensuring that you are getting the required medical care, having the required knowledge about what you should eat and avoid, and why certain foods are bad makes it easier to follow any diet.

Are you wondering how you can learn about all this? Well, you don't have to worry because this book has got you covered. This book will act as your guide every step of the way. It includes all the information required to understand what the renal diet means, how it functions, and all the dietary protocols it suggests. Apart from all this, you will learn about simple lifestyle changes and healthy habits that will help improve your overall health while promoting kidney functioning. Taking care of your kidneys is not as difficult or challenging as you once thought. Now that all the information is available at your fingertips, taking care of your health is easier than ever before. It is not just for the health of your kidneys, following this diet has other positive effects too. From reducing blood pressure to promoting weight loss and improving cardiovascular functioning, this diet has a lot to offer.

If you or anyone you know was recently diagnosed with a renal disorder or any other illness affecting the renal system, understand that you can improve your renal health. The responsibility of taking care of your physical health and wellbeing lies in your hands. The best way to ensure that your body functions effectively and optimally is by giving it the nutrients it needs. This means, paying attention to your diet is crucial. Following this diet not only improves kidney health but ensures the risk of any serious illnesses is also reduced. In a way, by following this diet, you will essentially be eating toward a healthier life and body.

Making a dietary change might not sound like much, but it is a significant change for your body and mind. This is especially true when you need to stop eating certain foods you are used to. The good news is you don't have to worry about consuming bland and flavorless meals. If you don't want to compromise on your tastebuds for the sake of health, this is the perfect book for you. In this book, you will discover several easy to cook, delicious, and nutritious recipes that can be whipped up within no time. You no longer have to dedicate hours in the kitchen cooking healthy meals.

You will also be introduced to practical steps and suggestions you can use to make healthy lifestyle changes. These changes will go a long way in maintaining the benefits obtained from the renal diet. Another important aspect of shifting to the renal diet is to understand that this is not a short-term solution or a quick fix. Instead, it is a long-term option for maintaining and improving the health of your kidneys. Even though there aren't any known cures for kidney diseases yet, the advances in modern medicine and science can be used to improve their functioning.

With a little patience, commitment, and consistency, you can work on improving your kidney health. If you are eager to learn more about all this, there is no time like the present to get started!

CHAPTER 1
About the Renal Diet

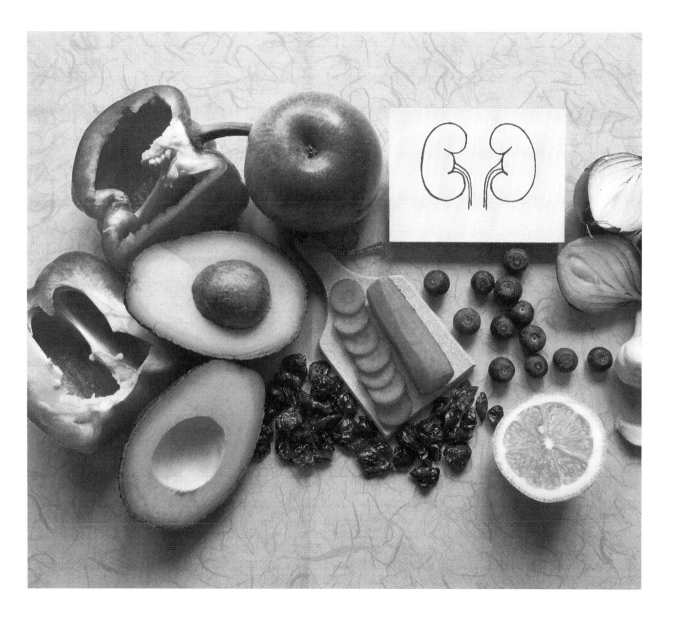

"Perfectly imperfect" is perhaps the best way to describe the mechanisms of the human body. Every cell has a specific function to play. Every tissue, organ, and system has clearly defined roles. Apart from their specific functions, they are intricately connected to ensure your body functions as intended. For instance, how you breathe not only affects the lungs, but regulates how oxygen reaches other parts of the body as well. Similarly, blood circulation has a significant effect on the functioning of all the organs present within. So, it is not surprising that what you eat and drink also has a significant effect on all the internal mechanisms.

THE ROLE OF KIDNEYS

To understand how the renal diet functions, it is important to understand the role played by kidneys. The primary function of the kidneys is blood filtration. All the blood circulating in your blood is filtered by the kidneys several times daily. Their primary aim is to ensure fluid balance while stabilizing the levels of electrolytes in the blood. Whenever blood reaches the kidneys, the waste present in it is removed and other elements in it, such as water, minerals, and salt, are adjusted. Once the blood is filtered, it goes back into circulation. All the waste is converted into urine that gets collected in the bladder and is ultimately drained out of the body through the urethra.

Kidneys are not only a part of the filtration and excretion systems, but have their own microsystems too. These systems contain millions of nephrons, or tiny filters, responsible for ensuring the optimal performance of kidneys. Kidneys play a vital role in blood filtration and are a crucial component of removing waste products building up in the body. Apart from this, they also release certain hormones responsible for controlling the production of red blood cells, regulating blood pressure, and releasing important vitamin D essential for maintaining the health of bones.

Any abnormality in the kidneys is categorized as kidney disease. Whether it's a marker such as a protein present in urine or something more systemic, they're all classified as kidney diseases. If anything reduces the function of kidneys for at least three months at a stretch, it is known as kidney disease. Kidney diseases are repetitive, consistent, and have a significant effect on the overall health of a person. Some common causes or risk factors associated with kidney diseases are high blood pressure, diabetes, and other congenital conditions. The good news is, improving kidney health and functioning is well within your control. Kidney disease doesn't have to prevent you from leading the life you desire. All it requires is a little consciousness of the heart and you can improve the health of your kidneys. The most important aspect of doing this is shifting to a healthy diet.

UNDERSTANDING THE RENAL DIET

The renal diet is created to support kidney functioning while reducing the progression of any kidney disease or disorder. It is designed to reduce the waste present in the blood by making certain changes to the foods and liquids you consume. When the kidneys cannot function as intended, their ability to filter or remove waste is also hampered. Excess buildup of waste in the blood results in an imbalance of electrolytes. By following the renal diet, all this can be reversed. Following the renal diet is one of the most important aspects of managing chronic kidney diseases. The renal diet ensures that there are no imbalances in the electrolytes, minerals, and fluid levels in your body. The renal diet not only improves the health and functioning of the kidneys but is good for your overall health too. The diet severely restricts your intake of processed and packaged foods, and replaces them with healthier and wholesome ingredients. Most of these ingredients are rich in antioxidants that reduce inflammatory responses and tackle inflammation. Apart from all this, they are known to reduce the risk of developing other chronic disorders including cardiovascular disorders, diabetes, and strokes.

Regulate Blood Pressure

When you follow the renal diet, your sodium intake automatically reduces. This, in turn, is believed to reduce your blood pressure levels. According to Miao Wang et al (2015), a low-sodium diet has a favorable effect on blood pressure levels. Since the renal diet automatically reduces your sodium intake, blood pressure levels will reduce this. High blood pressure is one of the leading health markers for a variety

of cardiovascular disorders. So, the renal diet helps improve the heart's health by reducing blood pressure.

Reduces Risk of Cancer

This diet is known to reduce the risk of certain types of cancer as well. Did you know that a high salt intake is associated with several types of cancer? A review of different studies showed that the risk of cancer increases by around 12% even if your daily salt intake increases by five grams (Xuexian Fang et al. 2015).On the other hand, a reduction in intake of salt is associated with a reduced risk of gastrointestinal cancer (Ian Johnson, 2015). Another benefit of following this diet is it will significantly reduce your consumption of red meats and processed meats. These two animal products are associated with an increased risk of different types of cancer. A combination of all these factors means you will not only be leading a healthier life but will reduce the risk of cancer too.

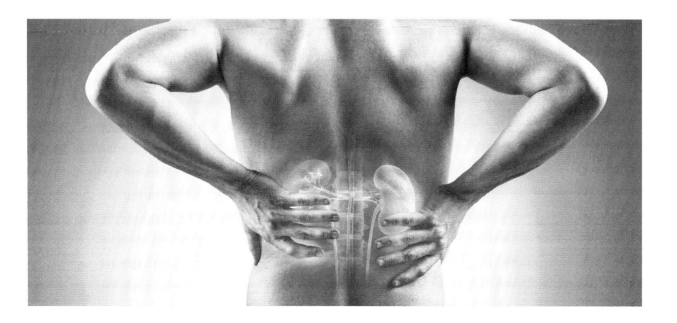

Better Nutrition

After you go through the renal diet food list discussed in this book, you will realize this diet is rich in wholesome and nutrient-dense ingredients. It also places a severe restriction on the consumption of processed and prepackaged foods. This diet will make you more mindful of the food choices you make. Instead of relying on strict calorie counting, the renal diet will increase your intake of healthy and whole foods that are important for improving your health. Such foods are rich in nutrients and healthy calories your body needs, unlike unhealthy or empty calories present in junk food. When your body gets the nourishment it needs, its ability to function effectively and efficiently also increases.

Weight Loss

The renal diet is low in sodium and includes healthy and high-quality protein. It also increases the consumption of low-carb vegetables. A combination of these factors and the drastic reduction in the intake of processed and prepackaged foods make it easier to lose weight. Being overweight or obese increases the strain on kidneys. By following this diet, your kidney health will improve. Apart from this, weight loss and maintenance also become easier. So, if you have been struggling to lose those extra pounds, you will see a positive change while following this diet. Apart from this, the high-quality protein suggested by this diet promotes satiety. If you are full, the chances of overeating will automatically reduce. In a way, this diet promotes weight loss without severe calorie restriction.

Healthy Protein

When you start following the renal diet, your consumption of healthy and high-quality protein increases. Protein is associated with better satiety levels when compared with unhealthy calories commonly found in most junk food. Protein suppresses appetite without making you feel deprived. Apart from this, it causes a temporary boost in metabolism. This means your body's ability to start utilizing the fat stored within improves. Metabolism is a simple chemical reaction through which the energy stored within is converted into a usable form and is immediately utilized. If you've been struggling to lose weight or have been asked to lose weight to improve your kidney functioning, increase consumption of high-quality protein.

A common side effect of kidney disease is loss of muscle mass. If you want to maintain your muscle mass, they must get the fuel they need. Well, the good news is that the amino acids present in protein act as building blocks for muscles. If you want to retain muscle or prevent muscle loss, ensure that you are consuming protein as per the recommendations of the renal diet. It also improves muscle recovery and growth. If you are exercising, even for a while, ensure that you rest after the exercise. During this, the protein you consume promotes the recovery of the muscles.

CHAPTER 2

Habits of People Winning the Disease

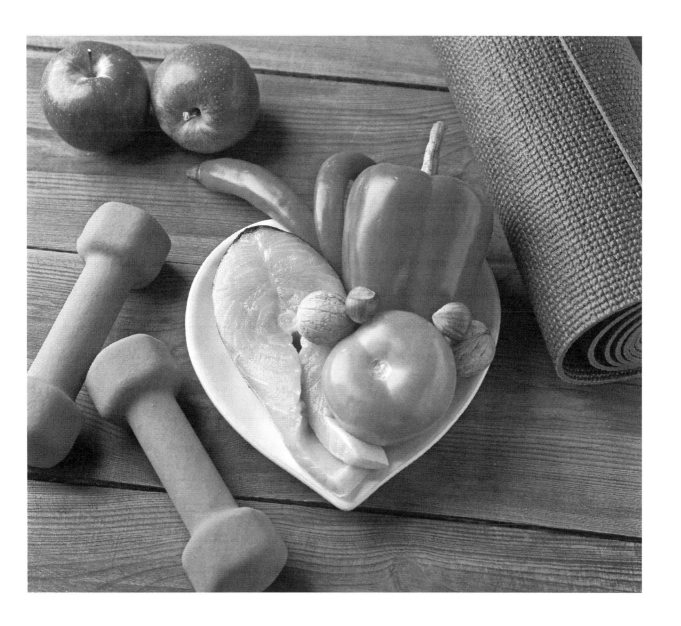

Living with kidney disease is not easy. That said, it's also important to understand that this disease shouldn't prevent you from living the life you want. If a kidney disorder or disease is getting in the way of your daily life, understand that you can adopt certain healthy lifestyle habits that will help fight it. In this chapter, let's look at healthy lifestyle changes that are associated with improving kidney health and winning the disease.

REGULAR EXERCISE

Exercising regularly is important for maintaining your overall health and fitness. Not just your physical well-being, even your mental health improves when you exercise regularly. You don't have to spend hours at the gym exercising. It is quite easy to set aside 30-minutes a day before exercise. Whether it is easy cardio, swimming, or any other physical activity you enjoy, ensure that you get your body moving. Even exercising for 30-minutes, three times a week has a positive effect on your overall well-being. This is one healthy lifestyle change that offers multiple benefits.

CONSUME A HEALTHY DIET

Consuming a healthy and wholesome diet is needed for ensuring that your body functions as intended. The diet you consume is the fuel that keeps you going. How can it perform properly if you don't give it the right fuel? Similarly, consuming a poor diet or a diet rich in unhealthy ingredients harms your overall health. One of the leading causes of obesity and weight gain is an unhealthy diet. Unfortunately, the modern diet is incredibly unhealthy as it relies mostly on processed and prepackaged foods that are devoid of nutrients. You don't have to count calories to follow a healthy diet. Instead, it's about consciously opting for wholesome and fresh ingredients instead of their processed counterparts.

Consuming a healthy diet makes it easier to maintain your healthy, ideal body weight. A host of chronic health problems such as high blood pressure, diabetes, and kidney failure are associated with obesity. Losing a couple of pounds will work wonders for your health, especially the health of kidneys.

REGULATE BLOOD SUGAR LEVELS

The risk of heart diseases and kidney failure increase due to diabetes. Diabetes is a condition where your body does not produce the insulin necessary for regulating blood sugar levels. It is also characterized by insulin sensitivity. This is a condition where the insulin produced is no longer enough to stabilize blood sugar levels. Diabetes is also a primary health marker for several chronic disorders. By managing your blood sugar levels, you can improve your kidney health.

HIGH BLOOD PRESSURE

High blood pressure or hypertension is associated with poor kidney health as well as an increased risk of heart diseases. When the pressure on the heart increases to ensure an optimal supply of blood is maintained to all cells, it is known as hypertension. A leading cause of hypertension includes poor diet, lack of sleep, and excess stress. By learning to manage your blood pressure level, you can improve kidney health.

NO SMOKING

Smoking is a silent killer. It reduces the flow of blood to the kidneys. Apart from it, it damages kidney function too. Smoking also harms the health of the lungs and heart, and increases inflammation. If you want to improve your kidney health, avoid smoking altogether. If you are in the habit of it, there is no time like the present to break free of it.

NO DRINKING

Alcohol is a known depressant. It not only causes mood swings but is incredibly harmful to your overall health. It is also rich in empty calories that are associated with weight gain. Apart from this, alcohol increases blood pressure. High blood pressure is harmful to your overall health, especially that of the heart and kidneys. So, avoid drinking.

AVOID USING OVER-THE-COUNTER PAIN-KILLERS

Using anti-inflammatory drugs and over-the-counter pain medications, such as ibuprofen and aspirin, reduces the flow of blood to the kidneys. Excess dependence on over-the-counter painkillers is, in general, harmful for your heart health too. If you want to improve your kidney health, avoid using them.

REDUCE SALT INTAKE

One important change that you must consciously make to your daily diet is to reduce salt consumption. A typical modern diet is rich in salt or sodium. Excess sodium consumption is associated with high blood pressure. It is also known to harm the functioning of kidneys, reduce electrolyte balance in the body, and also

results in water retention. By cutting down on your sodium intake, you can reverse all these conditions. Different spices and flavorings can be used for improving the flavor profile of meals you eat instead of relying on salt.

STAY HYDRATED

The importance of hydration cannot be overstated. From improving your skin health to ensuring your body functions properly, water is needed. Dehydration results in kidney damage by reducing the blood flow to them. If you don't drink sufficient water, it also increases the buildup of toxins present within. Those with kidney disorders need to be mindful of their fluid. So, talk to your healthcare provider before drastically reducing your fluid intake.

MANAGE STRESS

Learning to manage stress is good for your physical and mental health. It is also needed for maintaining your emotional wellbeing. Unfortunately, the modern world is filled with different stressors. Unless you learn to manage it, it will get the better of you. Also, there is no time like the present to get started with managing stress. Reducing stress and anxiety helps reduce blood pressure levels, which is good for the health of your kidneys and heart. Exercising regularly, getting sufficient sleep at night, and meditating daily are known to reduce stress.

By following all the different suggestions discussed in this section, you can improve your overall health and wellbeing and not just support your kidney health. Also, making these changes is not an overnight press. With a little conscious effort, patience, and consistency, improving your overall health becomes easier.

CHAPTER 3
Foods to Eat and Foods to Avoid

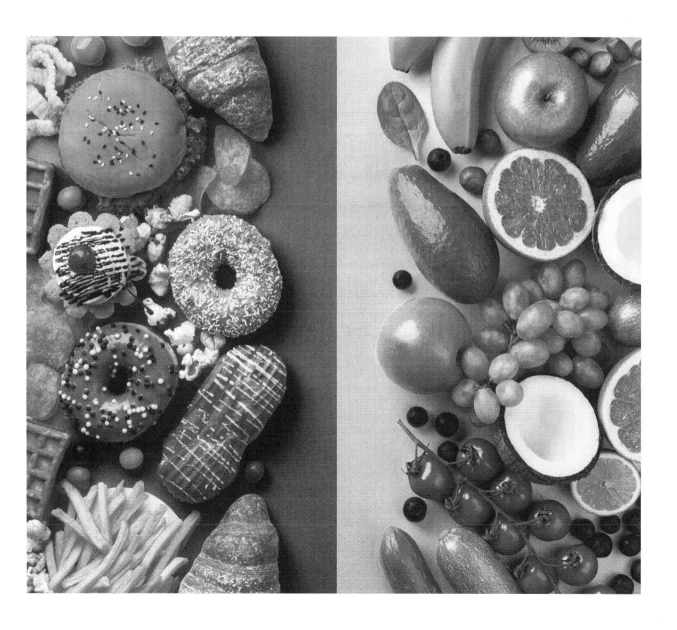

As mentioned, the first line of defense you can opt for to improve the functioning of your kidneys while slowing down the progression of a disease is to follow a healthy and wholesome diet. An important aspect of this is to understand the foods that you can eat and must avoid. When your kidneys are not functioning as intended, you must reduce the stress on them. The simplest way to do this is by avoiding certain foods that increase stress on them while increasing the consumption of foods that make things easier. Here is a list of foods that you can and cannot eat while following the renal diet.

FOODS TO EAT

To improve your overall health and strengthen kidney functioning, you need to consume foods that are low in sodium, potassium, and phosphorus. Apart from that, you must increase the consumption of high-quality protein and reduce fluid intake. Here is a list of foods you can eat while following the renal diet.

- You should opt for healthy proteins, such as chicken or turkey breast, skinless chicken and turkey, lean pork chop, salmon, trout, mackerel, shrimp, cod or tilapia, eggs, tofu, and unsalted nuts.

- You can opt for skimmed milk, plain yogurt, natural cheeses, and unsweetened soy, rice, or almond milk.

- Different whole grains that can be added to your diet are wild rice, brown rice, whole grain pasta, oatmeal, whole grain bread, unsweetened cereals, as well as unsalted pretzels and popcorn kernels.

- A variety of fresh and wholesome vegetables can be added to your daily diet such as bell peppers, asparagus, corn, cabbage, eggplants, zucchini, garlic, snow peas, broccoli, cucumbers, mushrooms, lettuce, celery, radishes, baby carrots, onions, green beans, and yellow beans.

- A variety of fresh fruits that strengthen and support the functioning of kidneys include apples, plums, berries, pineapples, grapes, pears, cherries, and peaches. You can also add all berries to your diet, as well as watermelon and dried cranberries.

- Different spices and flavorings can be added to enhance the flavor profile of your meals instead of depending on salt. All spices can be added and some flavorings you can use are garlic powder, chili powder, cumin, red wine vinegar, fresh lemons, limes, and olive oil.

- You must pay extra attention to all the beverages you drink because they increase fluid intake. You can opt for unsweetened tea and coffee, and clear diet soda. As a rule of thumb, it's always better to rely on water. Fresh juices can also be made with the fruits discussed above.

- You must stay away from repackaging processed foods that are rich in sodium, potassium, and phosphorus. That said, make it a point that you carefully need to read through the nutrition facts and list of ingredients whenever you purchase any of them.

NOTE: Certain processed and packaged foods can be added to your diet provided they are low in sodium, such as low-sodium canned fish, low-sodium cheese and natural cheeses, and prepackaged low-sodium seasoning and condiments. As much as possible, try to make the required condiments and seasonings at home. It hardly takes any time and it is worth the effort.

FOODS TO AVOID

In this section, let's look at all the different types of food you must avoid.

The first category of foods that you must avoid are those rich in sodium. You must stay away from all processed meats, such as deli meats, cured meat, smoked meats, and sausages. All preserved fish and seafood is also rich in sodium and, therefore, you must stay away from it. As a rule of thumb, all processed and pre-packaged foods are usually rich in sodium and you must stay away from it. That said, if the nutrition label mentions they are low in sodium, they can be consumed in regulated amounts.

- Deli meats
- Preserved fish and seafood
- Frozen or pre-packaged meals
- Canned food items such as soup or pasta
- Salted and canned beans
- Salted nuts and seeds
- Cheese, processed cheese products, and buttermilk
- Bread with extra salt, including dinner rolls and crackers
- Biscuits and pancake mix
- Pre-packaged or instant pasta, potatoes, and rice
- Canned vegetables and pre-packaged vegetable juices
- Salted vegetables or pickled vegetables
- Condiments such as ketchup, salsa, and mustard
- Dehydrated soup and broth
- Instant noodles
- Soy sauce
- Seasoning salts
- Marinades and pre-packaged salad dressings

- Salted butter and margarine, and pretty much all junk food you can think of

High potassium foods that you must avoid include the following:

- Cooked spinach, fried onions, okra, artichokes, broccoli, sweet potatoes, and beetroot
- Fruits such as bananas, oranges, honeydew melon, mangoes, pomegranate, coconut, prunes, pumpkins, and cantaloupe
- Milkshakes and buttermilk
- Baked and refried beans
- Legumes, including all lentils
- Nuts and seeds such as almonds, sunflower seeds, cashews, peanuts, pistachios, and butter made from them
- Whole grains and bran
- Granola bars and cereals
- Processed meats
- Vegetable juices
- Pre-packaged sauces
- Fruit juices made with the fruits discussed above and all processed fruit juices
- Ice creams, yogurt, frozen yogurt, and all chocolates

By avoiding the foods discussed in the section, your phosphorus intake will also reduce, which is desirable for improving your kidney health.

CHAPTER 4

Which Nutrients Need to Be Regulated

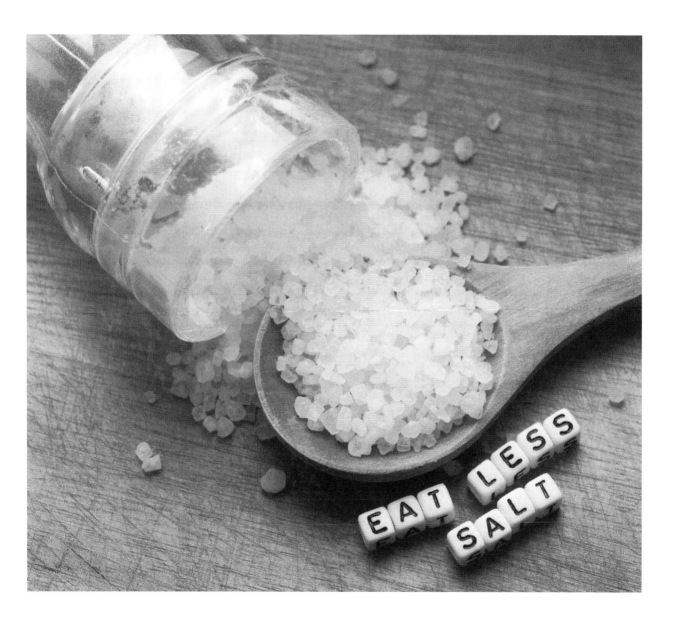

Making healthy food choices is crucial, but is even more important if you have any kidney disease. A well-balanced diet ensures that you have the required energy while slowing down the progression of kidney diseases. It means you must consume the right number of calories, proteins, vitamins, and minerals daily. To improve your kidney functioning while slowing down the progression of a kidney disorder or disease, regulate the intake of the nutrients discussed in this chapter.

SODIUM

One of the most important nutrients you must closely monitor is your sodium levels. When the kidneys are not functioning as intended, their ability to maintain water and sodium balance in the body is compromised. This is why you must restrict the intake of salt and fluids on the renal diet. Excess sodium consumption increases thirst, resulting in fluid restriction. The American Heart Association recommends that adults should not consume more than 2300 mg of sodium per day. This limit is further reduced to 1500 mg for anyone with hypertension or kidney disorders. It might sound like a lot, but to put things in perspective, 2300 mg sodium is present in a teaspoon of salt, including kosher and sea salt.

Sodium is an essential electrolyte. As an electrolyte, it's responsible for regulating the fluids that move in and out of the cells and tissues within the body. Apart from regulating blood pressure, it is responsible for maintaining the pH level of blood, muscle contraction, and elimination and retention of fluids. When there is excess sodium in your body, it increases thirst, results in swelling of extremities known as edema, increases blood pressure, and results in shortness of breath. Apart from this, it increases the risk of heart failure due to increased strain on the heart.

So, why is salt bad? Increased salt intake is associated with high blood pressure or hypertension. It, in turn, results in the stiffening and narrowing of blood vessels. In this condition, oxygen supply is reduced to organs, meaning the heart tries harder to pump the desired blood into the body. The increased stress on the heart increases blood pressure. Over a period, if this is left unregulated, high levels of blood pressure will compromise cardiovascular functioning. Hypertension also increases the stress on the kidneys. They increase the pressure on the filtering unit, which further impairs their ability to regulate fluid balance in the body (Silvio Borrelli et al 2020). This results in the worsening of any existing kidney disorders apart from harming cardiovascular health.

PHOSPHORUS

Phosphorus is an essential mineral that helps maintain the strength and health of bones and muscles. The small intestines are responsible for absorbing the phosphorus needed by the bones. All the extra phosphorus is removed by the kidneys. When the kidneys are unable to get rid of the extra phosphorus, it starts building up in the blood, and excess buildup of phosphorus in the blood results in the leaching of calcium from the bones, making them weak. When the phosphorus levels start increasing, it increases the presence of calcium deposits in the lungs, heart, kidneys, and blood vessels too. Increased intake of phosphorus not only worsens the progression of kidney diseases but increases the risk of cardiovascular diseases and mortality too (Isabel Rubio-Aliaga 2020). As with sodium and potassium, ensuring that your phosphorus levels are low is crucial while following the renal diet.

POTASSIUM

Potassium is one of the three crucial electrolytes the human body requires for its overall functioning. This mineral is commonly found in most foods and is needed for different functions. Potassium helps the heartbeat regularly and ensures the muscles are working as intended. The responsibility of regulating the levels of potassium in the body is controlled by the kidneys. When healthy, these organs know exactly how much potassium is needed. Any extra potassium is removed in the form of urine. When the kidneys are not functioning as intended, they cannot regulate the potassium level. Hyperkalemia is a condition where potassium levels are higher than needed. A direct relationship exists between increased intake of potassium and the risk of chronic kidney diseases (Kelly Picard et al 2020).

Hyperkalemia is associated with irregular heartbeat, slowing down of the pulse, excess weakness in the muscles, and increases the risk of heart attacks, stroke, and even death in extreme cases. Learning to limit your potassium intake is crucial for improving your kidney health. The first line of defense is to limit the consumption of foods that are rich in potassium. Apart from this, certain foods need to be avoided altogether because they are high in potassium.

PROTEIN

Protein is one of the three essential macronutrients your body needs for its overall functioning and health. Protein is needed for repairing tissue, building muscles, and fighting infections. If your kidneys are not functioning as intended, you must become mindful of your protein intake. It's not just about how much protein you consume, the quality of protein also matters. Protein results in the waste build-up in the blood. This, in turn, increases the stress on kidneys. Excess protein consumption or consuming poor-quality protein harms kidney health and functioning (Gang Jee Ko et al. 2017). Depending on the stage of kidney disorder or disease you are experiencing, the amount of protein you need to consume will vary. That said, as a rule of thumb, you should opt for high-quality, lean protein.

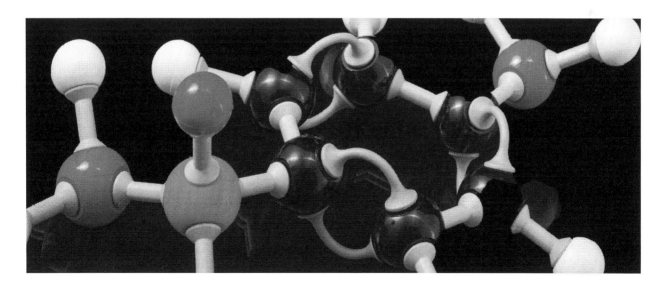

CHAPTER 5

Benefits of Exercise

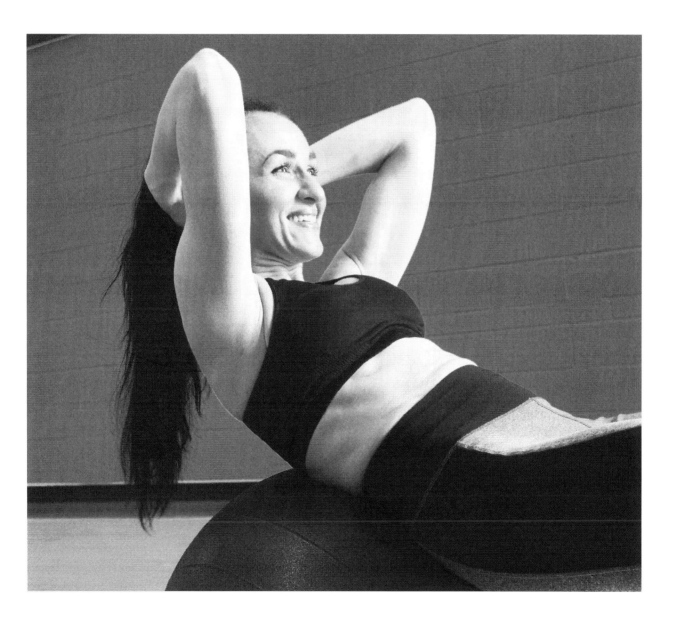

Previously, it was mentioned that adding exercise to your daily routine is important for improving your overall health and fitness levels. Most of us are guilty of leading sedentary lives with little or no exercise. If you are inactive, it increases the risk of developing several long-term chronic health problems, including strokes, heart diseases, diabetes, and depression. If you've been meaning to exercise, but never got around to doing it, there is no time like the present to make this healthy and important lifestyle change.

A wonderful thing about exercising is it is not just restricted to going to the gym. From playing sports, walking, running, jogging, and even dancing, there are different options available these days. If you don't want to go out, you can exercise within the comfort of your home as well! Depending on your existing fitness levels and the goals you want to achieve, the exercise pattern will differ. Also, don't forget to consult your healthcare provider about safe forms of exercise. The simplest way to get started is by walking or jogging regularly. This is the best cardio workout you can give your body.

Whenever you need to make a change, concentrating on all the benefits increases the motivation to make it. Exercising regularly is beneficial for kidney health. Exercising regularly reduces the risk of heart diseases and improves heart health, slows down the progression of kidney diseases, and improves other health markers (American Society Of Nephrology, 2014). In this section, let's look at all the different benefits you will gain by exercising regularly.

STRONG MUSCLES

Those struggling with kidney diseases usually feel tired and weaker than they used to. Muscles also start shrinking and wasting away. If you don't use your muscles regularly and ensure that you are keeping them strong, this will happen to anyone. However, this situation is further worsened if the kidneys are not functioning as intended. If they are not filtering out the toxins, your health is compromised. Forget about the notion that muscles are important only for bodybuilders and gym buffs. From moving around to climbing stairs and something as simple as getting out of bed, these movements are regulated by your muscles. They are also important for your usual health because they enable the stabilization of blood sugar. The best way to ensure that your muscles are healthy is by exercising regularly. Regular exercise is also associated with the prevention of diabetes and improved heart and kidney health.

IMPROVE HEART HEALTH

The risk of developing cardiovascular diseases increases when you have kidney disease. This means, focusing on improving your heart health is important. The simplest way to do this is by giving up smoking, regulating blood pressure and cholesterol levels, and managing blood sugar levels. The best way to do all this is by exercising regularly. Regular exercise is known to improve the health of blood vessels, reduce the risk of diabetes, lower blood pressure levels, and stabilize cholesterol levels. A combination of all these factors will automatically improve your cardiovascular functioning.

A HOLISTIC APPROACH TO HEALTH

One important benefit of regular exercise is it is needed for improving your mental, physical, and emotional well-being. We are exposed to different stressors daily. Whether it is the stress about your job, health, or finances, stress has become a constant companion in our lives. Tackling stress becomes easier when you start exercising regularly. Exercise is the best medicine for your body, mind, and soul. Exposure to constant stressors increases the production of a stress hormone known as cortisol. The best way to reverse this is by increasing the production of mood-enhancing hormones known as endorphins. Endorphins are also known as feel-good hormones. Exercise is the best way to increase the production of these helpful hormones.

BETTER ENERGY LEVELS

You need some energy to exercise. That said, your energy levels will improve when you start exercising regularly. It might be a little difficult initially, but once you get used to it, you will feel better and more energetic than ever before.

Ensure that you set aside some time daily for exercise. Find a type of physical activity that appeals to you and stick with it. By making exercise a conscious part of your daily life, your overall health will improve.

TIPS TO REMEMBER

Here are some simple and practical suggestions you should remember while exercising. These tips will ensure that your exercise routine is optimized for improved health.

When it comes to exercising, ensure that you are also spending some time outdoors. Whether it is running, jogging, biking, or even walking, spending some time away from being confined to the four walls of your home is a wonderful idea. This is good for your body and mind.

Whenever you are exercising, it's important to ensure that your body is thoroughly hydrated. Once you are aware of your required fluid intake, depending on your kidney health, ensure that you fulfill the quota daily. If you get dehydrated and are exercising, the chances of unknowingly injuring yourself increase.

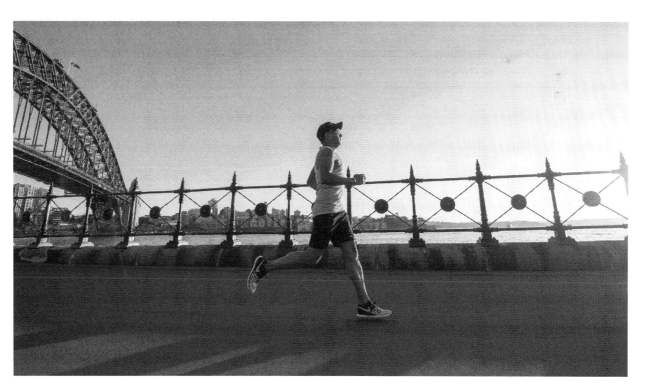

You must make a conscious decision of scheduling exercise into your daily routine. It is quite likely that you will not get to it if you keep telling yourself you will do it later. When you have a proper plan in place, sticking to the schedule also becomes easier. Even if it is only for 30 minutes, add it to your daily calendar. During this period, do not concentrate on anything else other than engaging in the physical activity of your choice.

You need to start thinking about exercise options outside the gym. Whether it is raking the leaves in your yard, gardening, or walking around the neighborhood, there are different options to choose from. Select an activity that makes you happy. The point is to engage in some form of physical activity or another. As mentioned, walking is perhaps the easiest form of exercise and it hardly takes any conscious effort. By using a pedometer or an app that helps track steps, you can make a note of how much you have walked. You can also establish simple workout goals and focus on achieving them.

If you are not used to exercising and are just getting started, maintaining your motivation levels is important. It is crucial that you do not get discouraged. There will be days when you feel energetic and days when you don't. Regardless of all this, ensure that you do not give up. It takes conscious effort, patience, and consistency to develop a habit. Once you get into the groove and start seeing the benefits it offers, your attitude toward exercise will change for the better.

Simple lifestyle changes can be made to ensure that your daily life encourages physical activity. For instance, instead of taking the elevator, you can take the stairs. Similarly, why don't you start walking or biking short distances instead of traveling by vehicle?

You need to let go of an all-or-nothing attitude when it comes to making exercise a part of your daily life. This attitude can prevent you from taking the first step. This mentality will make you believe that unless you exercise for 30 minutes, it doesn't count. There will be days when you only have 10 minutes to spare. Exercising for 10 minutes is better than not exercising at all. So, let go of this thinking pattern and, instead, focus on taking small steps.

CHAPTER 6
Preparing for the Diet

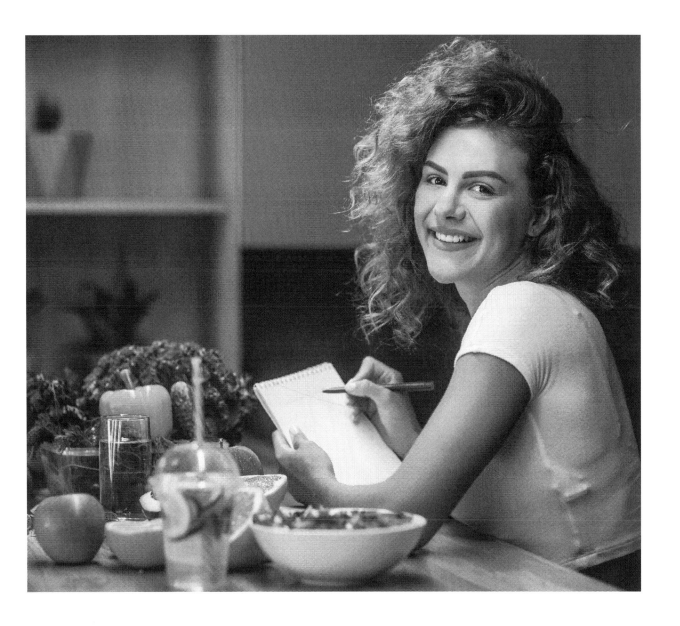

Making a dietary change might not sound like much. After all, it's just about adding and eliminating certain foods. It might sound simple but it is more complicated than most think. This is especially true if you are used to eating a certain way and your usual diet is rich in sugar, unhealthy carbs, empty calories, and processed foods. Most modern diets are rich in all this and are devoid of healthy and nutritious calories. Preparation is crucial for improving your chances of success and it is no different when it comes to starting the renal diet.

In this chapter, you'll be introduced to some simple suggestions that you must remember while preparing for the renal diet.

START WITH AN OBJECTIVE

Before you start the diet, ensure that you are aware of the objective or goal you are trying to achieve. Whether it is maintaining your existing level of health, losing weight for improving kidney health, or improving your overall well-being, there are different objectives. Ensure that you are aware of it. Without an objective, the chances of giving up on the diet increase. The objective must be personal and meaningful. After all, you will be making some significant changes, and unless the objective is meaningful, you cannot stick to the diet in the long run. As mentioned, following the renal diet is not a short-term solution. Instead, it's a long-term healthy dietary change.

GATHER THE REQUIRED INFORMATION

Before you start the diet, you must have all the required information. Without the required information, you cannot make the essential changes. From understanding the functioning of kidneys to what the renal diet means and all the benefits it offers, ensure that you have the needed information. Apart from the food list given in this book, ensure that you consult a healthcare provider about the same. Once you have the needed information, the reasons you should avoid certain foods and increase consumption of others becomes clear. The good news is all the information you need is given within this book!

KEEP AN OPEN MIND

Making a dietary change becomes difficult if you don't keep an open mind. In fact, making any change becomes difficult. So, concentrate on your mindset. A simple way to keep a positive mindset is by focusing on the objective you want to attain by following this diet. This is why you should always start with a specific objective. You will need to keep an open mind because certain foods that you thought were healthy will be eliminated while following the renal diet. For instance, most believe all types of protein are healthy. That said, while following the renal diet, you will be focusing more on high-quality protein instead of quantity.

One aspect of keeping an open mind about the diet you will be following is to focus on the foods you will be eating instead of the ones you won't. When you start concentrating too much on all the items you can no longer eat, the diet will feel restrictive. Instead, think of it as inclusive by focusing on all that you can eat. Also, once you start exploring the different recipes given in this book, your perception of diet food will change for the better. You will realize that following the renal diet is not only easy but includes the consumption of healthy, nutritious, and delicious meals.

A LITTLE FLEXIBILITY

Your diet must be a little flexible. If not, following it will become impossible. During the initial stages, making a dietary change is relatively easy because the motivation levels to follow it is high. With time, the motivation levels reduce. A simple way to ensure that you stay motivated is by adding some flexibility to your diet, which means your diet should not become so restrictive that you cannot enjoy your social obligations or usual lifestyle.

For instance, make allowances for what you can eat if you have to dine out or are traveling. The simplest way to ensure that you follow the diet is by preparing some renal diet-friendly snacks and carrying them with you at all times. The best way to ensure that your diet does not clash with social gatherings and special occasions is by planning.

SUPPORT SYSTEM

Before you start this diet, ensure that you have a support system in place. Your support system can include family members, spouse or partner, other loved ones, friends, or anyone else you can rely on and count on. It can include people present in your life, both online and offline. These days, multiple online options are available where you can interact with others who are in a similar situation as yours. Getting in touch with others who are experiencing what you are going through or have been through it, can be a refreshing experience. It will also make you feel that you are not alone.

Once you have a support system in place, you must talk to them about the dietary changes you are making and the reasons for the same. You cannot do it on your own. Also, there is no rea-son why you should do everything on your own. Relying a little on your loved ones, especially in your time of need, is a good idea. There will be days when following this diet will seem like an uphill battle or days when you don't want to keep going. On such days, your support system will give you the motivation required to keep going.

CLEAN YOUR PANTRY

Ensure that your pantry is stocked with renal diet-friendly ingredients. Apart from it, get rid of all foods that are prohibited by this diet. Remember, out of sight and out of mind is the best way to go about following a new diet. If you are constantly surrounded by temptations of foods that you should not eat, sticking to the diet becomes difficult. So, go through the food list discussed in the previous chapter, and stock your pantry with healthy ingredients.

MEAL PLANNING

Ensure that you spend sufficient time making a detailed meal plan for all the meals and snacks you can consume while following the renal diet. Meal planning not only ensures that you're following the diet but makes the diet easier too. The good news is you don't have to spend any extra time searching for renal diet-friendly recipes.

All the recipes you need are given in this book. Go through them, pick the recipes that you like, and start planning. An important aspect of meal planning is to make a note of different recipes you want to cook during the week. Once the plan is ready, shop for the required ingredients. Over the weekend, dedicate a couple of hours for meal prepping. Meal prepping is a healthy habit that makes cooking quite easy, especially when your weekday schedule is hectic. Some basic components of meal prep include cooking proteins, slicing up vegetables, and making sauces and other simple parts of a recipe. Another important benefit of meal planning is it ensures that your diet does not get boring and repetitive. If you have to eat the same food daily, it will become boring. This, in turn, will make it difficult to stick to the diet.

PORTION CONTROL

While following the renal diet, you do not have to worry about counting every calorie you consume. Calorie counting is not only restrictive but it can make you feel quite stressed too. Instead of calorie counting, practice the simple technique of portion control. Portion control is an effective and efficient means to ensure that you are consuming the right amount of healthy foods and are not going overboard. This also ensures that you are not overeating. This simple practice reduces the strain on your kidneys, helps maintain an ideal weight, and makes the food easier to digest. A combination of all these factors will help improve kidney functioning and health.

No matter what, you should never make significant changes to your diet and lifestyle without consulting a healthcare provider or dietitian. This is one step you should not overlook, especially while dealing with kidney disease. After all, your body cannot function effectively or efficiently if it doesn't get the required nourishment. This is why portion control should be practiced only according to the guidance of a healthcare provider. Before starting the diet, make sure that you consult a dietitian or a nutritionist and talk to them about your health condition and the goal you are trying to achieve. Consider their inputs and ensure that you fol-

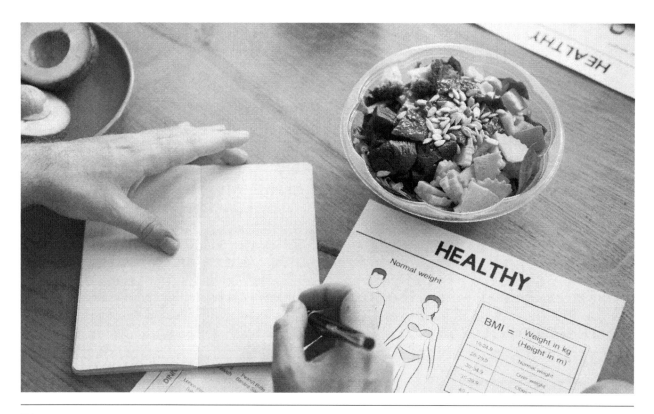

low a proper diet plan instead of a random one. After all, it is about improving your health and wellbeing. Erring on the side of caution is always better.

ASK FOR HELP

You are not alone. Please stop believing that you have to do everything on your own. If it feels like you need some help or support, reach out and ask for it. After all, help cannot be provided unless you ask for it. Let go of any stigma or shame associated with asking for help. Asking for help should be normalized because it's a sign of immense personal confidence and understanding. Knowing that you cannot do everything on your own is a strength. If you need any assistance with chores around the house, meal planning or prep, or any other assistance, reach out. After all, this is an example of times when your support system will come in handy.

START SMALL

You don't have to make all the changes in one go. Shifting to the renal diet is not a small change. It will take your body and mind some time to get used to it. Even if you are working on maintaining a positive mindset, it will not always be easy. This is why you must focus on taking small steps. If your usual diet is rich in foods that you can no longer consume, give your body and mind some time. Be patient with yourself. Be compassionate if you slip up or make any mistakes. Don't feel guilty if you eat food you know you're not supposed to. As long as you don't get into the habit of it or make a pattern out of it, it's all fine.

There will be days when you make a mistake or end up eating more than you are supposed to. On such days, treat it as an isolated incident and don't let it hamper your motivation to keep go-

ing. As long as you do this, it is fine. If there are different foods that you cannot eat, especially if they fall into low-quality protein, processed or packaged foods, or unhealthy captain sugars, you'll need to say goodbye to them. Eliminating such foods in one go is not easy. So, give yourself a couple of days to slowly transition to this diet. For instance, on the first day, you can cut out low-quality protein and replace it with high-quality ones. Similarly, avoid sugars and instead replace them with other foods. With a little creativity and planning, following this diet becomes easy. In this book, you will be introduced to a variety of renal diet-friendly recipes that will change your mind about dieting.

EXERCISE REGULARLY

Before you start this diet, ensure that you make time for exercising daily. You don't have to exercise for hours together. As mentioned in the previous chapter, even 30 minutes of exercise per day will improve your overall health and well-being. As long as exercise is part of your daily routine, your overall health will improve. Even on the days when you don't feel like doing it, ensure that you engage in some form of physical activity or the other. You cannot do this unless you schedule exercise into your daily routine.

KEEP TRACKING

You will need to make a conscious effort to track the progress you're making or any changes or fluctuations you notice in your overall health. It means you need to monitor your blood pressure, blood sugar, and weight closely. Apart from that, you should also pay extra attention to your lab results. When it comes to your health, you need to take a proactive role here. Set some reminders or alarms to ensure that you are regularly checking your blood pressure, blood sugar, and weight. These three factors play a significant role when it comes to influencing your kidney health. You can also use a spreadsheet for tracking your blood pressure and weight as per the dates. Ensure that you make a note of these health markers too.

Apart from this, ensure that you are showing up for all your doctor's appointments on time and without any delays. If you feel that something is amiss, chances are it is. If you are feeling more tired than usual after you've started exercising, take a break. Consult your healthcare provider immediately. If you notice any changes in your body, talk to the doctor about it. This applies to any changes you notice after shifting to the renal diet or an exercise routine. Also, do not make the mistake of believing that you need to wait until you get sicker to seek the required medical attention.

KEEP GOING

As mentioned, shifting to the renal diet is not an overnight process. It will take time and conscious effort. Meanwhile, you must ensure that you are not getting discouraged. At times, there might not be any significant change in your weight even after following the diet for a couple of weeks. In such instances, don't give up. Instead, look at the progress you are making. Each step taken in the right direction is a victory and it must be celebrated. Now is the time to be patient with yourself.

NOTE: We are all different and, therefore, our bodies are different too. Depending on the progression of the kidney disease and the stage of the disease, the diet you follow must change. There is no one-diet-fits-all approach when it comes to improving your kidney health. This is one of the reasons why you must consult your healthcare provider before making a dietary change. Whether it's the elimination or addition of certain ingredients, please contact your healthcare provider. Apart from this, it's important to understand that making a dietary change is good for your health.

CHAPTER 7

Breakfast Recipes

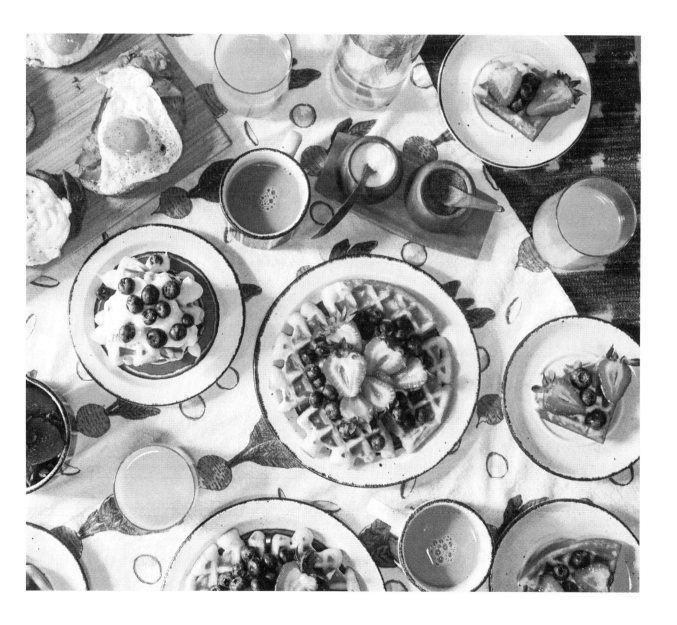

1. GREEN JUICE

Prep. time: 5 min | Cooking time: 0 min | Servings: 1

INGREDIENTS:

- 1 medium green apple
- ¼ cup chopped fresh pineapple
- 1 tablespoon lemon juice
- 1 small cucumber

NUTRITIONAL VALUES PER SERVING: ¾ CUP	
Calories	130
Fat	1 g
Carbohydrates	31 g
Protein	1 g
Sodium	4 mg
Potassium	366 mg
Phosphorus	46 mg

DIRECTIONS:

1. Core the green apple and cut into slices. Preferably, do not peel the apple.
2. Peel and chop fresh pineapple and measure out ¼ cup. Cut the cucumber into chunks. Remove the peel if desired.
3. Juice together green apple, pineapple, and cucumber in a juicer.
4. Pour into a glass. Stir in lemon juice.
5. Add some ice cubes or crushed ice if desired and serve.

2. HOT COCOA

Prep. time: 2 min | Cooking time: 2 min | Servings: 2

INGREDIENTS:

- 2 cups water
- 4 teaspoons granulated sugar
- 6 tablespoons whipped dessert topping
- 2 tablespoons unsweetened cocoa powder
- 4 tablespoons cold water

NUTRITIONAL VALUES PER SERVING	
Calories	72
Fat	3 g
Carbohydrates	13 g
Protein	1 g
Sodium	10 mg
Potassium	100 mg
Phosphorus	49 mg

DIRECTIONS:

1. Pour 2 cups of water into a saucepan. Place the saucepan over medium heat.
2. Meanwhile, combine cocoa powder, sugar, and 4 tablespoons cold water in a bowl.
3. When water starts boiling, turn off the heat.
4. Add the cocoa powder paste into the saucepan and stir until sugar dissolves completely.
5. Divide the hot cocoa into 2 cups.
6. Top each cup with 3 tablespoons of whipped dessert topping and serve.

3. APPLE CINNAMON MAPLE GRANOLA

Prep. time: 10 min | Cooking time: 50-60 min | Servings: 8

INGREDIENTS:

DRY INGREDIENTS:

- 1 z cups old fashioned oats
- ¼ cup dried, sweetened cranberries
- 1 ½ cups puffed rice cereal
- ½ package (from a 3.4 ounce package) baked apple chips
- ½ teaspoon ground nutmeg
- ¾ teaspoon ground cinnamon

WET INGREDIENTS:

- 2 tablespoons 100% pure maple syrup
- ¼ cup unsweetened applesauce
- 2 tablespoons melted coconut oil
- ¾ teaspoon vanilla extract

NUTRITIONAL VALUES PER SERVING: ½ CUP GRANOLA (without serving options)

Calories	162
Fat	6 g
Carbohydrates	25 g
Protein	2 g
Sodium	3 g
Potassium	107 mg
Phosphorus	70 mg

DIRECTIONS:

1. While you gather and prepare the ingredients, preheat your oven to 275°F. Prepare a baking sheet by lining it with a sheet of parchment paper.
2. Add old fashioned oats, dried cranberries, puffed rice cereal, and baked apple chips into a bowl and toss well.
3. Sprinkle ground nutmeg and ground ginger over the ingredients in the bowl. Toss well.
4. Combine applesauce, maple syrup, coconut oil, and vanilla extract in another bowl and whisk well. Drizzle this mixture over the granola mixture and toss until granola is well coated with the applesauce mixture.
5. Spread the granola onto the prepared baking sheet.
6. Place the baking sheet in the preheated oven and set the timer for about 50-60 minutes. Stir the mixture every 20 minutes and spread it once again after you stir.
7. Keep a watch on the granola after 40 minutes of baking as it can burn.
8. Take out the baking sheet from the oven and let it cool completely.
9. Transfer the granola into an airtight container and store at room temperature. It can last for a week.
10. You can serve it as it is or with some rice milk or any plant based milk that is recommended by your dietician or doctor. You can also add some berries or chopped apples if you are serving with milk.

4. CORNBREAD MUFFINS

Prep. time: 5-8 min | Cooking time: 15-20 min | Servings: 6

INGREDIENTS:

DRY INGREDIENTS:
- ½ cup plain cornmeal, white or yellow
- ½ cup all-purpose while flour
- 1 teaspoon baking powder
- ⅛ cup sugar

WET INGREDIENTS:
- ¼ cup liquid egg substitute
- 1 tablespoon unsalted melted butter or canola oil
- ½ cup unenriched rice milk

NUTRITIONAL VALUES PER SERVING: 1 MUFFIN	
Calories	124
Fat	3 g
Carbohydrates	23 g
Protein	3 g
Sodium	85 mg
Potassium	40 mg
Phosphorus	100 mg

DIRECTIONS:

1. While you are making the batter, preheat your oven to 400°F. Grease a muffin pan of 6 counts with some cooking oil spray. You can place disposable liners as well. This is optional.
2. Add all the dry ingredients into a bowl, i.e. cornmeal, all-purpose flour, baking powder, and sugar. Stir until well combined.
3. Add all the wet ingredients into another bowl, i.e. liquid egg substitute, butter, and rice milk. Whisk the mixture until smooth and well incorporated.
4. Add the flour mixture into the bowl of wet ingredients and stir until just incorporated, making sure not to overbeat. Distribute the batter among the 6 muffin cups in a muffin pan.
5. Place the muffin pan in the preheated oven and set the timer for 15-20 minutes or until done.
6. To check if the muffins are done, insert a toothpick in the center of the muffin. Pull the toothpick out. Check the toothpick to see if you can find any particles stuck on it. If you find any particles, you need to bake for some more time, maybe 5 minutes. If you do not see any particles stuck on the toothpick, the muffins are done and it is time to take the muffin pan out of the oven.
7. Let the muffins cool for a few minutes before taking them out from the pan. Serve them warm.

5. GREEN POWER SMOOTHIE

Prep. time: 10 min | Cooking time: 0 minutes | Servings: 2

INGREDIENTS:

- ½ cup unsweetened rice milk
- 2 cups baby kale
- Ice cubes, as required
- Lemon juice to taste (optional)
- ½ cup unsweetened dairy-free yogurt
- 2 apples
- 2 tablespoons melted coconut oil

NUTRITIONAL VALUES PER SERVING: 1 GLASS	
Calories	260
Fat	15.9 g
Carbohydrates	31.1 g
Fiber	5.8 g
Protein	1.4 g
Sodium	27 mg
Potassium	302.2 mg
Phosphorus	55.6 mg

DIRECTIONS:

1. Core the apples and peel them if desired. Cut into pieces.
2. Add apples into a blender along with yogurt, kale, ice cubes, and lemon juice into a blender.
3. Blend until you get a smooth mixture.
4. With the blender machine running, pour coconut oil in a thin stream through the feeder tube.
5. Divide the smoothie into 2 tall glasses and serve.

6. CRANBERRY MUFFINS

Prep. time: 15-20 min | Cooking time: 20 min | Servings: 24

INGREDIENTS:

DRY INGREDIENTS:
- 3 ½ cups all-purpose flour
- 4 teaspoons baking powder
- 14 tablespoons sugar
- ½ teaspoon salt

WET INGREDIENTS:
- 2 eggs
- ½ cup cooking oil
- 1 ½ cups cranapple juice
- 2 cups fresh or frozen cranberries

STREUSEL TOPPING:
- 6 tablespoons all-purpose flour
- 6 tablespoons brown sugar
- ½ teaspoon ground cinnamon
- 4 tablespoons unsalted butter

NUTRITIONAL VALUES PER SERVING: 1 MUFFIN	
Calories	187
Fat	7 g
Carbohydrates	29 g
Protein	3 g
Sodium	134 mg
Potassium	45 mg
Phosphorus	48 mg

DIRECTIONS:

1. While you are making the batter, preheat your oven to 400°F. Grease 2 muffin pans of 12 counts each, with some cooking oil spray. You can place disposable liners as well. This is optional.
2. Add all the dry ingredients into a bowl, i.e. all-purpose flour, baking powder, sugar, and salt. If you do not add the salt, the sodium in the recipe will reduce further. Stir until well combined. Make a well in the center of the mixture by pushing some of the flour mixture towards the sides of the bowl.
3. Coarsely chop some fresh or frozen and thawed cranberries and measure out 2 cups.
4. Crack the eggs into another bowl. Beat well. Add oil and cranapple juice, and whisk well.
5. Pour the mixture of wet ingredients into the bowl of flour mixture and stir until just combined, making sure not to overbeat. You may find some lumps in the batter but that is alright.
6. Add cranberries and fold gently.
7. Distribute the batter among the muffin cups in the prepared muffin pans. You should fill the batter up to ⊠ and no more than that.
8. To make streusel topping: Place all-purpose flour, brown sugar, and cinnamon in a bowl and stir until well combined.
9. Add butter and cut it into the flour mixture. You will have a crumbly mixture.
10. Scatter this mixture over the batter in the muffin cups.
11. Place muffin pans in the preheated oven and set the timer for 15-20 minutes or until done. If your oven is not large enough, bake the muffins in batches.
12. To check if the muffins are done, insert a toothpick in the center of the muffin. Pull the toothpick out and check to see if you can find any particles stuck on it. If you find any particles, you need to bake for some more time, maybe 5 minutes. If you do not see any particles stuck on the toothpick, the muffins are done and it is time to take the muffin pan out of the oven.
13. Let the muffins cool for a few minutes before taking them out of the pan.
14. Serve them warm.

7. SOUTHWEST BAKED EGG BREAKFAST CUPS

Prep. time: 10 min | Cooking time: 15 min | Servings: 6

INGREDIENTS:

- 1 ½ cups cooked rice
- 2 ounces green chilies, sliced
- ¼ cup skim milk
- ¼ teaspoon ground black pepper
- ¼ teaspoon ground cumin
- 2 ounces shredded cheddar cheese
- 1 ounce pimentos, drained, chopped
- 1 egg, beaten

NUTRITIONAL VALUES PER SERVING: 1 EGG CUP	
Calories	109
Fat	4 g
Carbohydrates	13 g
Fiber	0.5 g
Protein	5 g
Sodium	79 mg
Potassium	82 mg
Phosphorus	91 mg

DIRECTIONS:

1. While you are making the batter, preheat your oven to 400°F. Grease a muffin pan of 6 counts with some cooking oil spray. You can place disposable liners as well. This is optional.
2. Add rice, chilies, milk, pepper, cumin, egg, pimentos, and half the cheese into a bowl and stir until well combined.
3. Scoop the mixture into the muffin cups. Make sure the mixture is equally distributed.
4. Scatter remaining cheese on top.
5. Place the muffin pan in the preheated oven and set the timer for 15-20 minutes or until cooked and firm.

8. VEGETABLE SCRAMBLED EGGS

Prep. time: 10 min | Cooking time: 8-10 minutes | Servings: 1

INGREDIENTS:

- 2 whole eggs
- 1 ½ cup fresh spinach
- 2 tablespoons chopped bell pepper
- ½ cup chopped cauliflower
- 2 small cloves garlic, minced
- 2 tablespoons chopped onion
- ½ tablespoon coconut oil or avocado oil
- Pepper to taste
- A handful fresh parsley, chopped, to garnish

NUTRITIONAL VALUES PER SERVING: 1 PANCAKE	
Calories	240
Fat	16.6 g
Carbohydrates	7.8 g
Fiber	2.7 g
Protein	15.3 g
Sodium	15.3 mg
Potassium	605.2 mg
Phosphorus	253.6 mg

DIRECTIONS:

1. Crack eggs into a bowl. Add pepper and beat until frothy.
2. Place a skillet over medium heat. Add oil. When the oil is hot, add onion and bell pepper and cook until tender.
3. Add garlic and stir for a few seconds until you get a nice aroma.
4. Stir in the cauliflower and spinach. Lower the heat to medium-low. Cover the pan and cook for 3-4 minutes.
5. Stir in the eggs. Stir frequently until eggs are set.
6. Garnish with parsley and serve. If you want to reduce potassium in this dish, swap 2 whole eggs with 4 egg whites.

9. BELGIAN WAFFLES

Prep. time: 10-12 min | Cooking time: 3 minutes per waffle | Servings: 3

INGREDIENTS:

- 1 large egg, separate into white and yolk in 2 bowls
- ¼ teaspoon + ⅛ teaspoon baking soda
- 6 tablespoons 1% low fat milk
- 2 tablespoons unsalted butter, melted
- 3 tablespoons powdered sugar
- 1 tablespoon granulated sugar
- 1 cup cake flour
- 6 tablespoons sour cream
- 1 teaspoon vanilla extract

NUTRITIONAL VALUES PER SERVING: 1 EGG CUP	
Calories	367
Fat	15 g
Carbohydrates	50 g
Fiber	1 g
Protein	8 g
Sodium	204 mg
Potassium	151 mg
Phosphorus	121 mg

DIRECTIONS:

1. Plug in your waffle iron and preheat following the manufacturer's instructions.
2. Meanwhile, combine baking soda and cake flour in a mixing bowl.
3. Add sour cream, vanilla, and milk into the bowl of yolk and whisk well.
4. Pour butter and whisk well.
5. Set the hand mixer on medium speed and beat the egg white until soft peaks are formed.
6. Beat in the granulated sugar. Keep beating until stiff peaks are formed.
7. Add the milk mixture into the bowl of cake flour mixture and stir until just incorporated.
8. Add egg white and fold until just combined, taking care not to over mix.
9. Pour ⅓ of the batter (about ½ cup) into the preheated waffle iron. Close the lid and set the timer for 3 minutes or until the way you prefer it cooked.
10. Remove the waffle and sprinkle powdered sugar on top.
11. Cook the remaining 2 waffles in a similar manner.
12. Serve with your favorite toppings if desired.

10. BLUEBERRY SMOOTHIE

Prep. time: 5 min | Cooking time: 0 minutes | Servings: 2

INGREDIENTS:

- ½ cup frozen blueberries
- 2 teaspoons honey
- Ice cubes as required (optional)
- 2 cups rice milk
- 2 sprigs mint

NUTRITIONAL VALUES PER SERVING: 1 GLASS	
Calories	70
Fat	0.5 g
Carbohydrates	16.5 g
Fiber	1.1 g
Protein	0.3 g
Sodium	28.1 mg
Potassium	29.7 mg
Phosphorus	21.2 mg

DIRECTIONS:

1. Place blueberries, honey, rice milk, and mint in a blender. Blend for 30-40 seconds or until you get smooth puree.
2. Add ice if desired and blend once again.
3. Pour into 2 glasses and serve.

11. DENVER OMELET

Prep. time: 10 min | Cooking time: 5 min | Servings: 2

INGREDIENTS:

- ½ cup diced bell peppers of any color
- 1 ounce ham, diced
- 2 egg whites
- 2 large eggs
- 1 ounce extra-sharp cheddar cheese, shredded
- ½ cup chopped onion
- 2 teaspoons canola oil

NUTRITIONAL VALUES PER SERVING: ½ AN OMELET	
Calories	228
Fat	14 g
Carbohydrates	7 g
Fiber	0.9 g
Calories	17 g
Protein	5 g
Sodium	360 mg
Potassium	275 mg
Phosphorus	226 mg

DIRECTIONS:

1. Pour oil into a skillet and heat the oil over medium heat.
2. When oil is hot, add onion, bell pepper, and ham, and cook for a couple of minutes until the vegetables are tender.
3. Spread the mixture all over the skillet.
4. Crack the eggs into the bowl of whites and beat well. Add the egg mixture into the skillet and swirl the pan to spread the egg mixture.
5. Cook for a couple of minutes, until the egg sets. Using a spatula, loosen the omelet, around the edges.
6. Remove onto a plate. Scatter cheese on top. Cut into 2 halves and serve.
7. If you want to make 2 separate omelets, remove half the cooked mixture from the pan (after step 2). Pour half the egg mixture and cook the omelet.
8. Remove omelet from the pan. Add the retained cooked mixture back into the pan and cook the other omelet.

12. BLUEBERRY PANCAKES

Prep. time: 10 min | Cooking time: 3-5 min | Servings: 3

INGREDIENTS:

- ¾ cup sifted all-purpose flour
- 1 ½ tablespoons sugar
- 1 teaspoon baking powder
- ½ cup buttermilk
- 1 egg, lightly beaten
- 1 tablespoon unsalted margarine, melted
- ½ cup canned or frozen blueberries, rinsed
- Cooking spray

NUTRITIONAL VALUES PER SERVING: 2 PANCAKES	
Calories	223
Fat	6 g
Carbohydrates	35 g
Fiber	2 g
Protein	7 g
Sodium	196 mg
Potassium	128 mg
Phosphorus	100 mg

DIRECTIONS:

1. Combine all the dry ingredients in a bowl, i.e. flour, baking powder, and sugar.
2. Whisk in buttermilk, egg, margarine, and blueberries. Whisk until smooth. Initially, add 2 tablespoons of water and whisk.
3. Place a griddle or pan over medium heat. Spray the pan with a little cooking spray.
4. Pour ⅙ of the batter, about ⅓ cup. In about 40-60 seconds, bubbles will be visible on the pancake. Edges will begin to dry. Cook until the underside is golden brown.
5. Turn the pancake over using a spatula and cook the other side as well. Remove the pancake onto a plate and keep warm. Make the remaining 5 pancakes in a similar manner. Serve.

13. MUSHROOM AND RED PEPPER OMELET

Prep. time: 10 min | Cooking time: 3-5 minutes | Servings: 1

INGREDIENTS:

- ¼ cup chopped mushrooms
- ⅛ cup chopped red bell pepper
- 2 small eggs
- 1 tablespoon whipped cream cheese
- 1 tablespoon chopped onion
- 1 teaspoon butter
- ½ teaspoon Worcestershire sauce
- ⅛ teaspoon ground black pepper

NUTRITIONAL VALUES PER SERVING:	
Calories	199
Fat	15 g
Carbohydrates	4 g
Fiber	0.6 g
Protein	11 g
Sodium	276 mg
Potassium	228 mg
Phosphorus	167 mg

DIRECTIONS:

1. Add ½ teaspoon butter into a skillet and let it melt over medium heat.
2. Once butter melts, add onion and mushroom and cook until vegetables are tender.
3. Add bell pepper and mix well. Transfer the vegetables onto a plate.
4. Add ½ teaspoon butter and let it melt over low heat.
5. Meanwhile, crack eggs into a bowl. Add Worcestershire sauce and beat well.
6. Pour the egg mixture into the skillet and tilt the pan to spread eggs. Cook until the omelet is slightly set.
7. Scatter the cooked vegetables all over the omelet. Spoon the whipped cream cheese over the vegetables.
8. Once the eggs are cooked, slide a spatula around the edges of the omelet and slide onto a plate.
9. Sprinkle pepper over the omelet and serve.

14. CUCUMBER SAVORY PANCAKES

Prep. time: 15 min | Cooking time: 3-5 minutes | Servings: 2

INGREDIENTS:

- ¼ cup rice flour
- ⅛ cup peeled, grated potatoes
- ⅛ grated cucumber
- 1 tablespoon chickpea flour
- 1 green chili, very thinly sliced
- ½-⅔ cup water
- ¼ teaspoon salt
- 1 tablespoon finely chopped fresh cilantro
- Oil to cook the pancakes

NUTRITIONAL VALUES PER SERVING: 1 PANCAKE	
Calories	122
Fat	3.2 g
Carbohydrates	20.1 g
Fiber	2 g
Protein	2.8 g
Sodium	8.3 mg
Potassium	93.8 mg
Phosphorus	48.9 mg

DIRECTIONS:

1. Combine rice flour, potatoes, cucumber, chickpea flour, green chili, and cilantro in a bowl.
2. Add about ½ cup water initially and mix well. If the batter is too thick, add some more water and stir well. Place a griddle over medium heat. Let it heat. Spray the griddle with some cooking spray or brush some oil over the griddle.
3. Pour half the batter on the griddle and spread the batter on the skillet. Cook until the underside is golden brown. Turn the pancake over using a spatula and cook the other side as well.
4. Remove onto a plate and serve. Cook the other pancake similarly.

RENAL DIET COOKBOOK FOR BEGINNERS

15. FRUIT AND COTTAGE CHEESE OMELET

Prep. time: 15 min | Cooking time: 3-4 min | Servings: 2

INGREDIENTS:

- 4 eggs
- ½ cup low sodium cottage cheese
- Icing sugar to garnish (optional)
- 4 tablespoons water
- 1 cup canned fruit salad, drained

NUTRITIONAL VALUES PER SERVING: ½ AN OMELET

Calories	216
Fat	10 g
Carbohydrates	13 g
Fiber	1.3 g
Protein	19 g
Sodium	128 mg
Potassium	258 mg
Phosphorus	208 mg

DIRECTIONS:

1. Crack the eggs into a bowl. Add water and whisk well.
2. Place a nonstick pan over medium heat. Spray the pan with cooking spray.
3. Pour half the eggs into the skillet. Tilt the pan to spread the uncooked egg.
4. Cook until the omelet is nearly set and slightly moist in the center.
5. Slide a spatula around the edges of the omelet and loosen the omelet. Spread ¼ cup cottage cheese on the center of the omelet.
6. Place ¼ cup of the fruit salad over the cottage cheese. Fold the sides of the omelet over the filling.
7. Remove the omelet onto a plate.
8. Make the other omelet in a similar manner (steps 2-6).
9. Scatter ¼ cup fruit salad on top, over each omelet, and serve.

16. BAKED EGG CUPS

Prep. time: 10 min | Cooking time: 3-4 min | Servings: 2

INGREDIENTS:

- 4 eggs
- ½ cup low sodium cottage cheese
- Icing sugar to garnish (optional)
- 4 tablespoons water
- 1 cup canned fruit salad, drained

NUTRITIONAL VALUES PER SERVING: ½ AN OMELET

Calories	216
Fat	10 g
Carbohydrates	13 g
Fiber	1.3 g
Protein	19 g
Sodium	128 mg
Potassium	258 mg
Phosphorus	208 mg

DIRECTIONS:

1. Preheat your oven to 350°F. Grease a muffin pan of 6 counts with some cooking oil spray. You can place disposable liners as well. This is optional.
2. Cook bacon in a pan until crisp. Turn off the heat.
3. Remove bacon with a slotted spoon and place on a plate lined with paper towels.
4. When bacon cools, crumble into smaller pieces.
5. Add bacon and vegetables into a bowl and toss well.
6. Divide the vegetables equally into the muffin cups.
7. Whisk together eggs and pepper in another bowl. Divide beaten eggs among the muffin cups.
8. Place the muffin pan in the preheated oven. Set the timer for about 20-30 minutes or until the eggs are set well. Remove the muffin pan from the oven and let it cool for about 5-8 minutes. Loosen the edges of the muffins with a knife and remove the muffins. Serve immediately.

17. VEGAN COCONUT PANCAKES

Prep. time: 15 min | Cooking time: 20 min | Servings: 2

INGREDIENTS:

DRY INGREDIENTS:
- ½ cup + ⅛ cup sifted all-purpose flour
- ½ teaspoon baking soda
- 1 ½ tablespoons granulated sugar
- 1 teaspoon cream of tartar
- ½ teaspoon melted coconut oil + a little to fry the pancakes
- ¼ teaspoon vanilla or coconut extract

- 6 tablespoons canned coconut milk
- 2-4 tablespoons water

WET INGREDIENTS:
- 4 teaspoons maple syrup
- ½ cup canned pineapple pieces, drained
- ¼ cup unsweetened coconut flakes

NUTRITIONAL VALUES PER SERVING: 2 PANCAKES	
Calories	380
Fat	15.6 g
Carbohydrates	56.8 g
Fiber	2.5 g
Protein	5.7 g
Sodium	126.5 mg
Potassium	488.1 mg
Phosphorus	85.7 mg

DIRECTIONS:

1. Combine all the dry ingredients in a bowl, i.e. flour, baking powder, cream of tartar, and sugar.
2. Whisk in coconut oil, coconut milk, vanilla extract, and water. Whisk until smooth. Initially, add 2 tablespoons of water and whisk. If the batter is very thick, add a tablespoon or two of water.
3. Place a griddle or pan over medium heat. Add about ½ teaspoon of oil. Swirl the pan to spread the oil. Pour ¼ of the batter, about ¼ cup. In about 40-60 seconds, bubbles will be visible on the pancake. Edges will begin to dry. Cook until the underside is golden brown.
4. Turn the pancake over using a spatula and cook the other side as well. Remove the pancake onto a plate and keep warm. Make the remaining 3 pancakes in a similar manner.
5. To serve: Divide equally the maple syrup, pineapple, and coconut flakes among the pancakes and serve. Each serving has 2 pancakes.

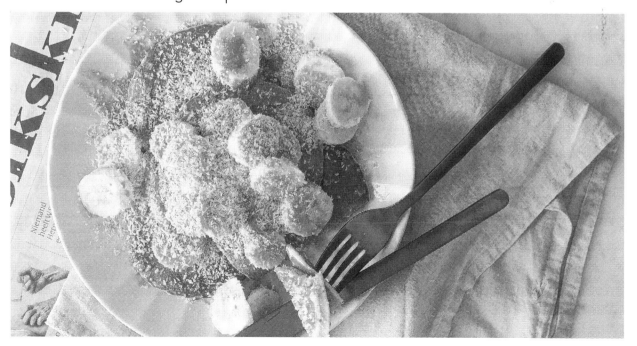

18. BANNOCK (LUSKINIKN)

Prep. time: 20 min | Cooking time: 35-45 min | Servings: 6

INGREDIENTS:

- 2 ½ cups all-purpose flour
- ¼ teaspoon + ⅛ teaspoon baking soda
- 1 ⅛ cups water
- 1 teaspoon cream of tartar
- ¼ cup + ½ tablespoon unsalted, non-hydrogenated margarine

NUTRITIONAL VALUES PER SERVING: ½ AN OMELET

Calories	267.4
Fat	9.1 g
Carbohydrates	40.1 g
Fiber	1.6 g
Protein	5.5 g
Sodium	84.9 mg
Potassium	140.89 mg
Phosphorus	57.66 mg

DIRECTIONS:

1. While you are preparing the dough, preheat your oven to 350°F.
2. Combine all-purpose flour, baking soda, and cream of tartar in a bowl.
3. Make a cavity in the center of the mixture. Pour water and ¼ cup margarine into the cavity and mix well until soft dough is formed. If the dough is too hard, add some more water.
4. Knead the dough in the bowl for about a minute.
5. Place the dough in a round cake pan. Pat the dough to fit the pan.
6. Score the bread on top, about ¼ inch deep, to make 4 equal portions.
7. Place the cake pan in the oven and bake for about 35-45 minutes or until golden brown on top.
8. Brush ½ tablespoon margarine on top. Cover the bannock with a kitchen towel for about 20-30 minutes. Cut along the scored part and serve.

19. SWEET CRUSTLESS QUICHE

Prep. time: 15 min | Cooking time: 50-60 min | Servings: 2

INGREDIENTS:

- 1 large egg
- 2 ⅔ tablespoons all-purpose flour
- ⅓ cup 2% milk
- Pepper to taste

FILLING:
- 4 teaspoons butter
- 1 medium apple
- 2 teaspoons brown sugar

NUTRITIONAL VALUES PER SERVING:

Calories	219
Fat	11.1 g
Carbohydrates	25.7 g
Fiber	2.5 g
Protein	5.5 g
Sodium	109.2 mg
Potassium	199.46 mg
Phosphorus	98.9 mg

DIRECTIONS:

1. While you are preparing the filling and batter, preheat your oven to 350°F.
2. Beat egg in a bowl. Add milk and whisk well. Add flour and beat until well combined. The batter may be a little lumpy.
3. To make filling: Core the apple and cut into slices. Peel the apple if desired. Combine apple, butter, and brown sugar in a saucepan and place the saucepan over medium-low heat. Cook until the sugar dissolves and the apples are well heated.
4. Grease a small cake pan with some cooking spray. Be generous with the oil or else the quiche may get stuck in the pan.
5. Spoon the filling into the cake pan. Spoon the batter over the filling.
6. Place the cake pan in the oven and set the timer for about 35-40 minutes or until golden brown on top. Cut into 2 equal portions and serve.

20. BRUSSELS SPROUT AND LEEK QUICHE

Prep. time: 20 min | Cooking time: 60 minutes | Servings: 4

INGREDIENTS:

CRUST:
- 6 tablespoons unbleached flour
- 2 ½ tablespoons unsalted butter, chilled, cut into cubes
- A tiny pinch sea salt
- 1-2 tablespoons ice water

FILLING:
- 1 tablespoon butter
- 3 ounces Brussels sprouts, thinly sliced
- 2 small eggs
- 3 tablespoons heavy cream
- ⅛ teaspoon freshly ground black pepper
- 2 ounces leek, white and light green parts, thinly sliced
- 1 tablespoon chopped tarragon
- 6 tablespoons whole milk
- 2 ounces goat cheese

NUTRITIONAL VALUES PER SERVING: ¼ QUICHE	
Calories	260
Fat	19 g
Carbohydrates	15 g
Fiber	1 g
Protein	8 g
Sodium	129 mg
Potassium	206 mg
Phosphorus	131 mg

DIRECTIONS:

1. While you are preparing the crust, preheat your oven to 350°F.
2. To make the crust: Add flour and salt into a bowl and stir.
3. Add butter into the flour mixture and cut it into it using a pastry cutter or your hands until you get crumbles of about the size of peas.
4. Add cold water, 1 tablespoon at a time, and mix well each time until the mixture comes together.
5. Dust your countertop with a little flour. Place dough on the countertop and knead the dough for a few minutes until a ball of the dough is formed.
6. Now roll the dough with a rolling pin to get a circle of about 6 inches diameter.
7. Place the dough in a small pie pan of about 4-5 inches diameter.
8. Place the dough in the pie pan and press it well onto the bottom as well as the sides.
9. Crimp the edges of the dough. Take a fork and pierce it at a few places on the bottom of the dough.
10. Lay a sheet of parchment paper over the dough. Place something heavy over the parchment paper in the pie pan. You can place some dried beans or chickpeas or anything else that you think is ok. This prevents the crust from rising.
11. Place the pie pan in the oven and set the timer for about 15-18 minutes, until the crust is half cooked.
12. Take out the pie pan from the oven and let it cool for some time.
13. Meanwhile, make the filling: Melt butter in a skillet over medium-high heat. Once butter melts, add Brussels sprouts, leek, and tarragon and mix well.
14. Lower the heat and cook until the vegetables are tender.
15. Turn off the heat.
16. Crack eggs into a bowl. Add milk and whisk well. Add goat cheese and pepper and whisk well.
17. Spread the brussels sprouts mixture over the half baked pie crust. Spoon the egg mixture over the vegetables.
18. Place the pie pan in the oven and set the timer for 30-40 minutes or until the eggs are cooked.
19. Cool for a few minutes. Cut into 4 equal wedges and serve.

21. FRESH BERRY FRUIT SALAD WITH YOGURT CREAM

Prep. time: 15 min | Cooking time: 0 min | Servings: 4

INGREDIENTS:

SALAD:
- 1 tablespoon honey
- ½ cup pitted, halved red cherries
- ½ cup raspberries
- ½ cup blackberries
- ½ cup blueberries

YOGURT CREAM:
- 1 cup Greek yogurt
- ½ tablespoon lemon juice
- 2 tablespoons honey
- flakes

NUTRITIONAL VALUES PER SERVING: ½ AN OMELET	
Calories	117
Fat	0.4 g
Carbohydrates	27 g
Fiber	3 g
Protein	3.7 g
Sodium	40 mg
Potassium	252 mg
Phosphorus	90 mg

DIRECTIONS:

1. **To make salad:** Place berries and cherries in a bowl and toss well. Drizzle honey and toss well. Chill until you serve (optional).
2. **To make yogurt cream:** Combine Greek yogurt, lemon juice, and honey in a bowl. Chill until use (optional).
3. **To serve:** Take 4 serving plates and divide the yogurt cream equally among the plates and spread it all over the center of the plate. Divide the salad among the plates and spread over the yogurt cream. Serve

22. ROOT HASH AND POACHED EGGS

Prep. time: 10 min | Cooking time: 8 min | Servings: 1

INGREDIENTS:

- ¾ tablespoon unsalted butter
- 1 scallion
- ½ small parsnip
- ½ small beet
- ½ medium carrot
- A pinch ground black pepper
- 1 medium cold egg
- 1-2 teaspoons white vinegar or apple cider vinegar

NUTRITIONAL VALUES PER SERVING:	
Calories	199
Fat	14 g
Carbohydrates	13 g
Fiber	4 g
Protein	7 g
Sodium	125 mg
Potassium	434 mg
Phosphorus	138 mg

DIRECTIONS:

1. Peel and grate the parsnip, beet, and carrot. Cut scallion into thin slices.
2. Place a small skillet over medium heat. Add butter and allow it to melt.
3. Once butter melts, add the root vegetables and stir-fry for a few minutes until the vegetables are tender.
4. Stir in scallion and black pepper and cook for a couple of minutes.
5. Transfer onto a plate.
6. While the vegetables are cooking, place a small saucepan with about 2 inches water, over high heat. Add vinegar.
7. When water begins to boil, break an egg into a bowl and slide the egg into the boiling water. Make sure you do not stir. Cover the saucepan, remove from heat, and let the egg rest in the hot water for 5 minutes.
8. Take out the egg from the saucepan and place over the root hash.
9. Serve.

23. CARROT PANCAKES

Prep. time: 15 min | Cooking time: 3-4 min | Servings: 6

INGREDIENTS:

- 3 cups skim milk
- 4 tablespoons unsalted butter
- 2 cups flour
- ⅛ teaspoon ground cinnamon
- ⅛ teaspoon ground nutmeg
- 4 medium carrots
- 2 teaspoons baking powder
- 2 tablespoons finely chopped walnuts
- 2 medium eggs
- 6 small medjool dates, pitted, finely chopped
- 1 teaspoon vanilla extract (optional)

NUTRITIONAL VALUES PER SERVING: 2 PANCAKES (without toppings)	
Calories	383
Fat	15 g
Carbohydrates	51 g
Fiber	4 g
Protein	11 g
Sodium	280 mg
Potassium	494 mg
Phosphorus	426 mg

DIRECTIONS:

1. Peel the carrots and chop into pieces. Add carrots into a blender along with butter, flour, spices, baking powder, eggs, and milk.
2. Blend the mixture until smooth and well combined. Transfer the batter into a bowl.
3. Stir in dates and walnuts.
4. Place a griddle or pan over medium heat. Spray the pan with a little cooking spray.
5. Pour about ⅓ cup of batter on the pan. In about 40-60 seconds, bubbles will be visible on the pancake. Edges will begin to dry. Cook until the underside is golden brown.
6. Turn the pancake over using a spatula and cook the other side as well. Remove the pancake onto a plate and keep warm.
7. Make the remaining 11 pancakes in a similar manner. You can store the leftover pancakes in an airtight container in the refrigerator. Reheat and serve. It can last for about 4 days.
8. Serve with some toppings of your choice.

24. WATERMELON SMOOTHIE

Prep. time: 10 min | Cooking time: 0 minutes | Servings: 1

INGREDIENTS:

- 1 cup chopped, deseeded watermelon, frozen
- Few mint leaves
- ½ medium cucumber
- ½ stalk celery, sliced
- Juice of ½ a lime

NUTRITIONAL VALUES PER SERVING: 1 GLASS	
Calories	143
Fat	0.9 g
Carbohydrates	35.2 g
Fiber	3.4 g
Protein	4.1 g
Sodium	41.1 mg
Potassium	887 mg
Phosphorus	115 mg

DIRECTIONS:

1. Once you chop the fresh watermelon, place on a tray and freeze until firm.
2. Place watermelon, mint, cucumber, celery, and lime juice in a blender.
3. Blend until you get smooth puree.
4. Pour into a tall glass. Garnish with a mint leaf or place a watermelon wedge on the rim of the glass. This piece of watermelon should not be frozen.

25. BERRYLICIOUS SMOOTHIE

Prep. time: 5 min | Cooking time: 0 min | Servings: 1

INGREDIENTS:

- 2 tablespoons cranberry juice cocktail
- ¼ cup frozen, unsweetened blueberries
- ¼ cup frozen, unsweetened raspberries
- ¼ teaspoon powdered lemonade
- ⅓ cup firm, silken tofu
- ½ teaspoon vanilla extract

NUTRITIONAL VALUES PER SERVING: 1 GLASS	
Calories	115
Fat	3 g
Carbohydrates	18 g
Fiber	1 g
Protein	6 g
Sodium	14 mg
Potassium	223 mg
Phosphorus	80 mg

DIRECTIONS:

Place berries, cranberry juice cocktail, powdered lemonade, vanilla extract, and tofu in a blender. Blend for 35-50 seconds or until smooth. Pour into a tall glass. Serve.

26. PEACH RASPBERRY SMOOTHIE

Prep. time: 5 min | Cooking time: 0 min | Servings: 1

INGREDIENTS:

- ⅓ cup frozen raspberries
- 2 ½ tablespoons tofu
- ⅓ cup unfortified almond milk
- ⅓ medium peach, sliced
- 1 teaspoon honey

NUTRITIONAL VALUES PER SERVING: 1 GLASS	
Calories	129
Fat	3.2 g
Carbohydrates	23 g
Fiber	4.8 g
Protein	6.3 g
Sodium	53 mg
Potassium	261 mg
Phosphorus	72 mg

DIRECTIONS:

Place raspberries, tofu, almond milk, peach, and honey in a blender and blend until you get smooth puree. Pour into a tall glass and serve.

27. BERRY BEET SMOOTHIE BOWL

Prep. time: 10 min | Cooking time: 0 min | Servings: 1

INGREDIENTS:

- ½ medium beet
- ½ cup frozen raspberries
- ½ cup frozen mango chunks
- ½ cup unsweetened rice milk
- 1 tablespoon slivered almonds
- ¼ cup mixed berries of your choice
- ½-1 teaspoon maple syrup

NUTRITIONAL VALUES PER SERVING: 1 GLASS	
Calories	188
Fat	5.7 g
Carbohydrates	33.4 g
Fiber	8.2 g
Protein	4.6 g
Sodium	127.3 mg
Potassium	537.5 mg
Phosphorus	95.9 mg

DIRECTIONS:

1. Peel and grate the beet. Place beet in a blender. Add raspberries (thaw them if frozen), mango, maple syrup, and rice milk and blend until you get thick puree.
2. Pour into a bowl. Scatter mixed berries and almonds on top and serve.
3. If you want lower potassium, replace mango with frozen pineapple.

28. ACAI BERRY SMOOTHIE BOWL

Prep. time: 10 min | Cooking time: 0 min | Servings: 1

INGREDIENTS:

- ½ packet unsweetened frozen acai
- 6 tablespoons plain 2% low-fat Greek yogurt
- ¼ cup unsweetened rice milk
- ½ cup frozen mixed berries, unsweetened
- ½ teaspoon chia seeds
- ⅛ fresh pear, chopped
- 1 tablespoon blueberries
- 1 tablespoon raspberries

NUTRITIONAL VALUES PER SERVING: 1 GLASS	
Calories	192
Fat	4 g
Carbohydrates	28 g
Fiber	7.2 g
Protein	11 g
Sodium	82 mg
Potassium	349 mg
Phosphorus	140 mg

DIRECTIONS:

Break the frozen acai into smaller pieces and add into a blender.

Add yogurt, rice milk, mixed berries, and chia seeds into the blender and blend thick until creamy.

Pour into a bowl. Scatter blueberries, raspberries, and pear on top and serve.

29. SUMMER VEGETABLES OMELET

Prep. time: 15 min | Cooking time: 3-4 minutes per omelet | Servings: 2

INGREDIENTS:

- ½ cup frozen corn kernels, thawed
- 6 tablespoons chopped green onions
- ⅔ cup chopped zucchini
- ½ teaspoon pepper or ½ teaspoon extra spicy Mrs. Dash seasoning
- 2 whole eggs
- 4 large egg whites
- ¼ cup water
- 2 ounces shredded low fat sharp cheddar cheese

NUTRITIONAL VALUES PER SERVING:	
Calories	187
Fat	6 g
Carbohydrates	11 g
Fiber	1.6 g
Protein	22 g
Sodium	270 mg
Potassium	352 mg
Phosphorus	218 mg

DIRECTIONS:

1. Spray a nonstick pan with cooking spray and place it over medium heat.
2. Add zucchini, corn, and green onions and cook until the vegetables are crisp as well as tender. Transfer on to a plate. Clean the pan and place it back over medium heat.
3. Whisk together eggs, whites, water, and seasoning in a bowl.
4. Spray with cooking spray and let the pan heat.
5. Pour half the egg mixture into the pan. When the edges begin to set, lift the edges of the omelet to let the uncooked egg go onto the bottom of the pan.
6. When the eggs are cooked around the edges and slightly uncooked in the center, loosen the omelet around the edges with a spatula.
7. Place half the vegetable mixture on one half of the omelet. Scatter half the cheese over the vegetables. Fold the other half of the omelet over the filling and cook for a couple of minutes.
8. Remove onto a plate and serve.
9. Make the other omelet in a similar manner (steps 4-8).

30. SAVORY BREAKFAST PIZZA

Prep. time: 20 min I Cooking time: 20-30 min I Servings: 8

INGREDIENTS:

PANCAKE:
- 1 cup Bob's Red Mill 1-to-1 gluten-free baking flour
- ¼ teaspoon kosher salt
- ¼ teaspoon ground nutmeg
- 1 teaspoon baking soda
- ½ teaspoon ground pepper
- ¼ teaspoon red pepper flakes
- 6 ounces water
- 4 tablespoons lemon juice
- 6 large eggs
- 5 ounces whole milk
- 4 tablespoons unsalted butter

FILLING:
- 2 tablespoons oil
- 4 teaspoons minced garlic
- 1 cup thinly sliced asparagus
- ¼ cup chopped fresh parsley
- ½ cup diced red onion
- 7 ounces fresh shiitake mushrooms, diced
- ½ cup shredded sharp cheddar cheese
- ½ teaspoon fresh lime zest

TO SERVE (OPTIONAL):
- Maple syrup
- Balsamic glaze

NUTRITIONAL VALUES PER SERVING: 1 WEDGE (without serving options)

Calories	275
Fat	16 g
Carbohydrates	21 g
Fiber	2 g
Protein	9 g
Sodium	328 mg
Potassium	241 mg
Phosphorus	167 mg

DIRECTIONS:

1. While you are preparing the batter, preheat your oven to 350°F.
2. To make pancake: Combine all the dry ingredients in a bowl, i.e. flour, salt, nutmeg, pepper, red pepper flakes, and baking soda.
3. Crack eggs into another bowl. Add milk, water, and lemon juice and whisk well.
4. Add butter into a large, round baking dish. Place the dish in the oven for a few minutes until butter melts.
5. Take out the dish from the oven and brush the butter all over the bottom of the pan.
6. Spoon the batter into the pan and bake for 25-30 minutes or until slightly brown around the edges and dry on top.
7. Meanwhile, make the filling: Pour oil into a pan and place it over medium heat. Add onions and sauté until translucent.
8. Stir in the garlic and cook for a few seconds until you get a nice aroma.
9. Stir in the mushrooms. Stir often for about 3 minutes. Now add asparagus and mix well.
10. Once asparagus turns bright green, turn off the heat.
11. Scatter the vegetable mixture over the baked pancake. Sprinkle cheese on top.
12. Place the baking pan in the oven and continue baking for a couple of minutes until the cheese melts.
13. Cut into 8 equal wedges and serve.

31. POHA

Prep. time: 10 - 12 min I Cooking time: 10 min I Servings: 6

INGREDIENTS:

- 3 cups thick flattened rice (poha)
- ½ teaspoon turmeric powder
- 4 tablespoons peanuts
- 2-4 green chilies, split
- 4 tablespoons of cooking oil like sunflower etc.
- 1 cup finely chopped onions
- 1 ¼ teaspoons black mustard seeds

- A handful fresh or dried curry leaves
- 2 teaspoons sugar or to taste
- Juice of a lemon
- 1 teaspoon salt

TO GARNISH:
- A handful fresh cilantro, chopped
- A handful grated fresh coconut

NUTRITIONAL VALUES PER SERVING:

Calories	264
Fat	17 g
Carbohydrates	25 g
Fiber	3 g
Protein	5 g
Sodium	442 mg
Potassium	145 mg
Phosphorus	82 mg

DIRECTIONS:

1. Rinse the flattened rice a few times in water. Drain in a colander. Let it rest for 15 minutes.
2. Meanwhile, chop the onion and measure out a cup of onions.
3. Place a heavy pan over medium heat. Add peanuts and dry roast them until they have a crunch.
4. Transfer the peanuts onto a plate and let it cool.
5. Pour oil into the pan and let it heat. Once hot, add mustard seeds. The mustard seeds will start spluttering.
6. Add onion, curry leaves, and green chilies and cook until onion turns translucent. Add turmeric powder and salt and stir for about 5 – 6 seconds.
7. Add flattened rice and mix well. Cover the pan and lower the heat. Cook for about 8-10 minutes, stirring every 2-3 minutes.
8. Add lemon juice and peanuts, stir. Transfer into a serving bowl. Garnish with cilantro and coconut and serve.
9. Store leftovers in an airtight container in the refrigerator. You can reheat in a microwave and serve. In case you are storing, it is recommended to store the peanuts in a separate container and mix it up when you reheat.

32. CHIA SEED PUDDING

Prep. time: 5 min | Cooking time: 0 min + chilling time | Servings: 2

INGREDIENTS:

- ¼ cup chia seeds
- 2 tablespoons maple syrup
- ¾ cup rice milk
- ½ teaspoon vanilla extract
- ⅛ teaspoon ground cinnamon

NUTRITIONAL VALUES PER SERVING: ½ CUP (without fruits)	
Calories	187
Fat	8.1 g
Carbohydrates	25.7 g
Fiber	9.1 g
Protein	4.3 g
Sodium	11.1 mg
Potassium	153.5 mg
Phosphorus	230.5 mg

DIRECTIONS:

1. Place chia seeds, maple syrup, rice milk, vanilla extract, and cinnamon in a bowl.
2. Stir well and cover the bowl. Chill for 4-8 hours.
3. Divide the pudding into 2 bowls. Add some renal diet friendly fruits if desired and serve.

33. CHICKEN RICE PORRIDGE OR CONGEE

Prep. time: 10 min | Cooking time: 30 min | Servings: 10

INGREDIENTS:

- 4 cups rice
- 20 cups water + extra to dilute if necessary
- 6 green onions, thinly sliced
- 4 bone-in chicken breasts, skinless
- 2 inches fresh ginger, peeled, julienne cut
- 2-3 teaspoons sesame oil
- 2 teaspoons soy sauce
- Pepper to taste
- 2 teaspoons salt

NUTRITIONAL VALUES PER SERVING	
Calories	200
Fat	5 g
Carbohydrates	24 g
Fiber	1 g
Protein	12 g
Sodium	430 mg
Potassium	250 mg
Phosphorus	191 mg

DIRECTIONS:

1. Rinse the rice well, a few times and place in a large pot. Pour 20 cups of water and place the pot over medium heat. Cover the pot with a lid.
2. When water starts boiling, add chicken and stir. When water starts boiling once again, add salt and pepper and cook until rice and chicken are cooked. Whenever the chicken cooks, take it out of the pot and place on your cutting board.
3. If the congee is very thick, add some water to dilute.
4. When cool enough to handle, shred chicken and add it back into the pot. Mix well.
5. Stir in ginger and sesame oil and remove from heat.
6. Serve in bowls garnished with green onions, soy sauce, and a generous sprinkle of pepper.
7. Store leftovers in an airtight container in the refrigerator. To serve: Reheat in a pan or microwave adding a little water and serve.

34. CHOCOLATE GRANOLA

Prep. time: 10 min | Cooking time: 10 min | Servings: 5

INGREDIENTS:

- 1 cup rolled oats
- 0.6 ounce almonds, sliced
- 2 teaspoons chia seeds
- 2 tablespoons maple syrup
- ⅓ teaspoon vanilla extract
- 0.8 ounce unsalted pecans
- 2 tablespoons unsweetened cocoa powder
- 0.8 ounce sweetened dried cherries
- 1 ⅓ tablespoons melted coconut oil

NUTRITIONAL VALUES PER SERVING: ½ CUP (without serving options)	
Calories	178
Fat	9 g
Carbohydrates	23 g
Fiber	4 g
Protein	4 g
Sodium	3 mg
Potassium	153 mg
Phosphorus	114 mg

DIRECTIONS:

1. While you gather and prepare the ingredients, preheat your oven to 350°F. Place a sheet of parchment paper over a baking sheet.
2. Place oats, nuts, chia seeds, and cocoa powder in the food processor bowl. Give short pulses until roughly chopped.
3. Place the chopped mixture into a bowl. Add cherries and toss well.
4. Pour oil, maple syrup, and vanilla extract and toss well.
5. Transfer the mixture on the baking sheet. Spread the mixture evenly over the baking sheet.
6. Place the baking sheet in the oven and set the timer for 20 minutes. Stir the mixture after 10 minutes of baking. Keep a watch over the granola after 15 minutes of baking, as the granola can burn.
7. Let the granola cool completely on your countertop.
8. Add the cooled granola into an airtight container.
9. You can serve it with toppings of your choice, but of course renal diet friendly.

35. FERMENTED BUCKWHEAT PORRIDGE

Prep. time: 5 min + fermenting time | Cooking time: 12-15 min | Servings: 2

INGREDIENTS:

- ⅔ cup green buckwheat groats
- 2-4 tablespoons kefir
- 4 cups water

NUTRITIONAL VALUES PER SERVING: (without toppings)	
Calories	204
Fat	2 g
Carbohydrates	41 g
Fiber	6 g
Protein	8 g
Sodium	33 mg
Potassium	261 mg
Phosphorus	117.6 mg

DIRECTIONS:

1. Grind the buckwheat groats into a powder using the coffee grinder.
2. Add into a saucepan. Add water and kefir and stir well. Cover and place it on your countertop. Let it remain on your countertop overnight.
3. Just before breakfast, place the saucepan over medium heat. Stir constantly until the porridge is thick.
4. Turn off the heat and divide into 2 bowls. Serve with toppings of your choice if desired.

36. CHIA, COCONUT, AND BUCKWHEAT PORRIDGE

Prep. time: 10 min | Cooking time: 8-10 min + chilling time | Servings: 2

INGREDIENTS:

- ½ cup buckwheat groats (do not use kasha)
- 1 ½ cups coconut milk or rice milk, unsweetened
- 1 teaspoon vanilla extract
- A dash of salt
- 2 tablespoons chia seeds
- ½ cup water or more if required
- ⅛ teaspoon ground cinnamon

NUTRITIONAL VALUES PER SERVING (without optional toppings)	
Calories	406
Fat	22 g
Carbohydrates	47 g
Fiber	12 g
Protein	11 g
Sodium	10 mg
Potassium	398 mg
Phosphorus	247 mg

DIRECTIONS:

1. Add buckwheat groats and chia seeds into a bowl. Pour vanilla extract, water, and coconut milk and mix well.
2. Keep the bowl covered with cling wrap and keep it in the refrigerator overnight.
3. The next morning, transfer the buckwheat mixture into a saucepan. Cook the mixture over medium heat until the thickness you desire is achieved. Stir occasionally.
4. Divide into 2 bowls. Serve with renal diet friendly toppings if desired.

37. PARAGUAYAN CHEESE BREAD (CHIPA ARGOLLA)

Prep. time: 15 min | Cooking time: 25 min + chilling time | Servings: 16

INGREDIENTS:

- ½ cup unsalted butter, softened
- 6 ounces mozzarella cheese, grated
- 1 teaspoon anise seeds
- 1 cup cornstarch (fine cornmeal/corn flour)
- 1 ⅓ cups milk
- 6 medium eggs
- 2 ounces parmesan cheese, grated
- ½ teaspoon salt
- 2 cups cassava flour

NUTRITIONAL VALUES PER SERVING	
Calories	216
Fat	12 g
Carbohydrates	21 g
Fiber	2 g
Protein	7 g
Sodium	222 mg
Potassium	131 mg
Phosphorus	139 mg

DIRECTIONS:

1. While you are preparing the dough, preheat your oven to 420°F.
2. Place butter and eggs in the mixing bowl of the stand mixer. Fix the dough attachment.
3. Beat for about a minute. Add mozzarella and parmesan cheese and mix well. Add anise seeds and mix well. Combine salt and milk in a bowl and pour into the mixing bowl.
4. Combine cassava flour and cornstarch in another bowl and add into the mixing bowl. Mix until well incorporated. Dust your countertop with some flour. Place dough on the countertop and knead well for a few minutes and soft dough is formed.
5. Divide the dough equally into 16 equal portions and shape into balls. Place on a baking sheet. Cover the dough balls with a kitchen towel and place in the refrigerator for about 20 minutes.
6. Take a ball of dough and roll it into a rope of about 6 inches in length and ½ inch in diameter.
7. Hold the ends of the rope together to make a circle. Press the ends together so that it is well sealed.
8. Line 2 large baking sheets with parchment paper. Place the bread on the baking sheet. Repeat this process with the remaining dough balls. Leave a gap of about 3 inches between the breads on the baking sheet.
9. Bake them in batches for about 20-25 minutes or until light golden brown on top.

38. LEMON BERRY BREAD

Prep. time: 15 min I Cooking time: 40-50 min I Servings: 24

INGREDIENTS:

CRUST:
- 3 cups all-purpose flour
- 1 ⅓ cups granulated white sugar
- 2 teaspoons baking powder
- 8 egg whites
- 2 cups fresh blueberries
- ⅔ cup canola oil
- 4 tablespoons lemon extract
- 1 cup 1% low-fat milk
- 2 tablespoons grated lemon zest

FILLING:
- 1 ½ cups powdered sugar
- 2 tablespoons grated lemon peel

NUTRITIONAL VALUES PER SERVING: 1 SLICE	
Calories	212
Fat	15 g
Carbohydrates	34 g
Fiber	0.8 g
Protein	3 g
Sodium	54 mg
Potassium	66 mg
Phosphorus	68 mg

DIRECTIONS:

1. While you are preparing the batter, preheat your oven to 350°F. Grease 2 loaf pans (9 x 5 inches each) with some oil.
2. Mix together flour and baking powder in a mixing bowl.
3. Whisk together sugar, oil, milk, egg whites, and lemon extract in another bowl.
4. Add the flour mixture into the bowl of wet ingredients and stir until just incorporated, making sure not to over mix.
5. Add blueberries and lemon zest and fold gently.
6. Divide the batter equally among the loaf pans. Place the loaf pans in the oven and set the timer for 40-50 minutes.
7. To check if the bread is done, you insert a toothpick in the center of a loaf. Pull the toothpick out. Check the toothpick to see if you can find any particles stuck on it. If you find any particles, you need to bake for some more time, maybe 5 minutes. If you do not see any particles stuck on the toothpick, the loaves are done and it is time to take out the loaf pans from the oven.
8. Let the loaves cool for a few minutes before taking them out from the pan.
9. Meanwhile, make the glaze: Add powdered sugar and lemon juice into a small saucepan. Place the saucepan over medium heat and stir often until sugar dissolves completely.
10. Pierce the top of the loaves with a toothpick at different spots (leave a gap of 1 inch between the holes). Divide the glaze equally and spoon the glaze all over the loaves.
11. Cool completely. Cut each loaf into 12 slices each and serve.
12. Store leftovers in an airtight container at room temperature for 2-3 days or in the refrigerator for 5-6 days.

39. CRANBERRY NUT BREAD

Prep. time: 20 min | Cooking time: 1 hour and 10 minutes | Servings: 20

INGREDIENTS:

- 2 cups sugar
- 1 teaspoon baking soda
- 3 teaspoons baking powder
- 4 cups all-purpose flour
- 3 cups fresh cranberries, halved
- 2 large eggs
- 2 teaspoons grated orange zest
- ½ cup chopped walnuts
- 1 cup cranberry juice or apple juice
- 4 tablespoons margarine
- 4 tablespoons hot water

NUTRITIONAL VALUES PER SERVING: 1 SLICE	
Calories	214
Fat	5 g
Carbohydrates	40 g
Fiber	1.3 g
Protein	4 g
Sodium	143 mg
Potassium	85 mg
Phosphorus	58 mg

DIRECTIONS:

1. While you are preparing the batter, preheat your oven to 350°F. Grease 2 loaf pans (9 x 5 inches each). Line them with parchment paper as well.
2. Sift together flour, baking soda, and baking powder in a mixing bowl.
3. Sprinkle sugar all over the flour mixture and stir well.
4. Crack eggs into a bowl. Add cranberry juice, margarine, and orange zest and whisk well.
5. Pour the egg mixture into the bowl of flour mixture and mix until just incorporated, making sure not to over beat. Add walnuts and cranberries and stir. Add hot water and stir.
6. Divide the batter among the loaf pans.
7. To check if the bread is done, insert a toothpick in the center of a loaf. Pull the toothpick out. Check the toothpick to see if you can find any particles stuck on it. If you find any particles, you need to bake for some more time, maybe 5 minutes. If you do not see any particles stuck on the toothpick, the loaves are done and it is time to take out the loaf pans from the oven.
8. Let the loaves cool for a few minutes before taking them out from the pan.
9. Place the loaves on a wire rack to cool. Cut each loaf into 8 equal slices and serve. Store leftovers in an airtight container at room temperature for 2-3 days or in the refrigerator for 5-6 days.

40. VANILLA CREPES

Prep. time: 10 min | Cooking time: 1-2 minutes per crepe | Servings: 4

INGREDIENTS:

- ½ cup milk
- 2 teaspoons vanilla extract
- 2 teaspoons sugar
- 5 teaspoons melted butter
- 1 egg yolk
- ½ cup all-purpose flour
- A pinch salt

NUTRITIONAL VALUES PER SERVING: 1 CREPE (without toppings)	
Calories	142
Fat	6.7 g
Carbohydrates	15.9 g
Fiber	0.4 g
Protein	3.3 g
Sodium	146 mg
Potassium	71.7 mg
Phosphorus	83 mg

DIRECTIONS:

1. Combine yolk, milk, and vanilla in a bowl. Add flour, salt, sugar, and butter and whisk until smooth.
2. Place a nonstick pan or a crepe pan over medium-high heat. Brush some oil over it.
3. Take ¼ of the batter and pour it on the heated pan. Tilt the pan to spread the batter.
4. Cook for about 45 seconds. Turn the crepe over and cook for about 20 seconds.
5. Remove onto a plate and serve with renal diet friendly toppings or fillings.
6. Cook the remaining crepes similarly.

41. SOUTHERN STYLE GRITS

Prep. time: 2 min | Cooking time: 25-30 min | Servings: 1

INGREDIENTS:

- 3 tablespoons stone-ground grits
- 3 tablespoons milk
- ½ tablespoon butter
- Pepper to taste
- ½ cup water
- A pinch salt

NUTRITIONAL VALUES PER SERVING: 2 MUFFINS	
Calories	93
Fat	6 g
Carbohydrates	7 g
Fiber	0.7 g
Protein	2 g
Sodium	158 mg
Potassium	71 mg
Phosphorus	45 mg

DIRECTIONS:

1. Add grits, milk, water, salt, and ¼ tablespoon butter into a heavy bottom saucepan.
2. Place the saucepan over low heat and cook for about 20-30 minutes, until it gets thick.
3. Stirring very often or constantly.
4. Turn off the heat. Add ¼ tablespoon butter and some pepper to taste.
5. Mix well and serve.

42. HOMEMADE MUESLI

Prep. time: 15 min | Cooking time: 10 minutes | Servings: 8

INGREDIENTS:

- 4 cups grains rolled oats and wheat bran
- 1 ½ cups nuts/seeds such as sliced almonds, walnuts, flaxseeds, sunflower seeds, pumpkin seeds, sesame seeds, chia seeds or a mixture
- ½ cup dried fruit such as chopped apricots, raisins, apples, figs, goji berries, or a mixture
- Honey
- Yogurt

NUTRITIONAL VALUES PER SERVING	
Calories	150
Calcium	20 g
Protein	36 g
Sodium	70 mg
Potassium	45 mg
Phosphorus	96 mg

DIRECTIONS:

1. Place the grains, nuts and seeds in a frying pan and heat. Stir frequently until they look lightly toasted but not brown. Transfer them in a large bowl and let them cool.
2. Stir in the dried fruits. Put the muesli in an airtight container and store at room temperature for up to a 3 weeks. You can serve topped with the yogurt if you like.

43. VERY BERRY BREAD PUDDING

Prep. time: 10 min | Cooking time: 50 min | Servings: 5

INGREDIENTS:

- 4 cups cubed challah bread
- 1 cup heavy cream
- ¼ cup sugar
- ½ tablespoon grated orange zest
- Non dairy whipped cream to serve (optional)
- 3 eggs, beaten
- 6 ounces frozen mixed berries, thawed
- 1 teaspoon vanilla extract
- ¼ teaspoon ground cinnamon

NUTRITIONAL VALUES PER SERVING (without whipped cream)	
Calories	392
Fat	23 g
Carbohydrates	36 g
Fiber	2.2 g
Protein	9 g
Sodium	231 mg
Potassium	134 mg
Phosphorus	172 mg

DIRECTIONS:

1. Grease a baking dish with some oil. Also preheat your oven to 375°F.
2. Crack eggs into a bowl. Add cream, sugar, vanilla, orange zest, and cinnamon and whisk until well combined.
3. Add breadcrumbs and berries and mix well. Transfer the mixture into the baking dish.
4. Keep covered with foil and place it in the oven. Set the timer for about 45-50 minutes.
5. Uncover after about 30 minutes of baking and continue baking until pudding is set.
6. Serve with whipped cream if desired.

44. FRUITY MUFFIN AND BREAD PUDDING

Prep. time: 15 min | Cooking time: 25 min | Servings: 3

INGREDIENTS:

- ½ cup whole-milk yogurt
- 2 tablespoons light brown sugar
- ⅛ teaspoon ground nutmeg
- 1 medium ripe plum, pitted, quartered
- ½ medium very ripe pear, cored, peeled, diced
- ¼ teaspoon ground ginger
- A tiny pinch sea salt
- 2 large eggs, lightly beaten
- 1 tablespoon raisins
- 5 ounces ciabatta bread or French bread, cut into about 1 inch cubes
- 1 tablespoon powdered sugar to garnish

NUTRITIONAL VALUES PER SERVING: 2 MUFFINS	
Calories	272
Fat	7 g
Carbohydrates	44 g
Fiber	3 g
Protein	10 g
Sodium	307 mg
Potassium	257 mg
Phosphorus	148 mg

DIRECTIONS:

1. While you are making the batter, preheat your oven to 375°F. Grease a muffin pan of 6 counts with some cooking oil spray, place disposable liners as well (optional).
2. Blend together yogurt, nutmeg, ginger, salt, plum, eggs, and brown sugar in a blender until smooth.
3. Combine bread, pear, and raisins in a bowl. Pour the blended mixture over the bread.
4. Distribute the mixture among the 6 muffin cups in a muffin pan. Press the mixture down into the muffin cups.
5. Place the muffin pan in the preheated oven and set the timer for 20-25 minutes or until golden brown on top.
6. Let the muffins cool for a few minutes before taking them out from the pan. Loosen the edges of the muffins by running a knife around the edges of the muffins. Serve them warm.

45. BUCKWHEAT PANCAKES

Prep. time: 10 min | Cooking time: 3-4 min per pancake | Servings: 2

INGREDIENTS:

- ¾ cup + ⅛ cup unsweetened rice milk
- ¼ cup all-purpose flour
- ½ cup buckwheat flour
- 1 teaspoon baking powder
- ½ tablespoon sugar
- ½ teaspoon vanilla extract
- 1 teaspoon white vinegar
- 1 small egg
- 1 tablespoon unsalted butter, divided

NUTRITIONAL VALUES PER SERVING: ½ CUP (without serving options)	
Calories	281
Fat	9 g
Carbohydrates	43 g
Fiber	4 g
Protein	7 g
Sodium	167 mg
Potassium	241 mg
Phosphorus	199 mg

DIRECTIONS:

1. To make buttermilk: Add rice milk and vinegar into a bowl and stir. Set aside for 5 minutes.
2. Whisk in the eggs and vanilla.
3. Combine the dry ingredients in a bowl, i.e. buckwheat flour, all-purpose flour, baking powder, and sugar. Pour the egg mixture into the bowl of dry ingredients and mix until just combined, making sure not to over mix.
4. Place a griddle or pan over medium heat. Add ½ tablespoon butter and allow it to melt.
5. Pour ½ of the batter on the griddle. In about 40-60 seconds, bubbles will be visible on the pancake. Edges will begin to dry. Cook until the underside is golden brown.
6. Turn the pancake over using a spatula and cook the other side as well. Remove the pancake onto a plate and keep warm. Make the other pancake in a similar manner. Serve.

46. BUCKWHEAT CREPES

Prep. time: 5 min + resting time | Cooking time: 1-2 min per crepe | Servings: 4

INGREDIENTS:

- 1 ¼ cups water
- ¼ teaspoon salt
- ¾ cup buckwheat flour
- Oil to cook
- ¼ teaspoon baking soda (optional but recommended)

NUTRITIONAL VALUES PER SERVING: 1 CREPE (without toppings)	
Calories	75
Fat	1 g
Carbohydrates	16 g
Fiber	2 g
Protein	3 g
Sodium	230 mg
Potassium	130 mg
Phosphorus	89 mg

DIRECTIONS:

1. Whisk together water, salt, baking soda, and buckwheat flour in a mixing bowl. You should have a smooth batter.
2. Rest the batter for about 30 minutes.
3. Mix well once again.
4. Place a nonstick pan or a crepe pan over medium-high heat. Brush some oil over it.
5. Take ¼ of the batter, about ½ cup, and pour it on the heated pan. Tilt the pan to spread the batter.
6. Cook for about 45 seconds. Turn the crepe over and cook for about 20 seconds.
7. Remove onto a plate and serve with renal diet friendly toppings or fillings.
8. Cook the remaining crepes similarly.

47. SUMMER SAUSAGE

Prep. time: 5 min I Cooking time: 50-60 min I Servings: 5

INGREDIENTS:

- ½ pound ground beef
- 1 teaspoon mustard seeds
- ¼ teaspoon ground black pepper
- ¼ teaspoon garlic powder
- ¼ teaspoon onion powder
- ⅛ teaspoon kosher salt
- ¾ teaspoon liquid smoke
- ½ tablespoon Nature Restore celery juice powder
- 1 teaspoon Orrington Farms low-sodium beef broth powder
- 1 ounce water

NUTRITIONAL VALUES PER SERVING	
Calories	113
Fat	8 g
Carbohydrates	1 g
Fiber	0 g
Protein	12 g
Sodium	104 mg
Potassium	146 mg
Phosphorus	89 mg

DIRECTIONS:

1. Place a rack on a broiler pan. Preheat your oven to 400°F.
2. Combine meat, spices, salt, liquid smoke, celery juice powder, water, and broth powder in a bowl.
3. Give a cylindrical shape to the mixture. Wrap it up in 2 sheets of foil and place on the rack.
4. Pour some water in the broiler pan, around 2 cups. Place the broiler pan along with the rack in the oven and set the timer for about 40-50 minutes or until the internal temperature of the meat in the center of the log shows around 165°F.
5. Do not unwrap for 30 minutes. Unwrap now and let it cool for another 8-10 minutes. Cut into 5 equal slices and serve.

48. CHEESY GRITS

Prep. time: 5 min I Cooking time: 10-15 min I Servings: 1

INGREDIENTS:

- ½ cup water
- A pinch salt (optional)
- 1 teaspoon unsalted butter
- ¼ cup 2% low-fat milk
- 1 teaspoon minced basil
- 3 tablespoons white or yellow grits
- 2 tablespoons shredded sharp cheddar cheese

NUTRITIONAL VALUES PER SERVING	
Calories	214
Fat	10 g
Carbohydrates	23 g
Fiber	1.2 g
Protein	8 g
Sodium	268 mg
Potassium	133 mg
Phosphorus	142 mg

DIRECTIONS:

1. Combine water, salt, and milk in a heavy pan and place the pan over medium-high heat.
2. When the mixture starts boiling, stir in the grits.
3. Lower the heat and cover the pan partially. Stir frequently and cook for about 5 minutes if you are using quick cooking grits or 8-10 minutes if you are using old-fashioned grits.
4. Turn off the heat. Add cheese and stir.
5. Serve hot garnished with basil.

49. APPLE OATMEAL CUSTARD

Prep. time: 5 min | Cooking time: 3 min | Servings: 2

INGREDIENTS:

NUTRITIONAL VALUES PER SERVING: ½ CUP	
Calories	248
Fat	8 g
Carbohydrates	33 g
Fiber	5.8 g
Protein	11 g
Sodium	164 mg
Potassium	362 mg
Phosphorus	240 mg

- ⅔ cup quick-cooking oatmeal
- 1 cup almond milk
- 1 medium apple, cored, finely chopped
- 2 large eggs
- ½ teaspoon ground cinnamon

DIRECTIONS:

1. Add eggs and almond milk into a microwave safe bowl and whisk well.
2. Add oats, apple, and cinnamon and stir well.
3. Place the bowl in the microwave and cook on high for 3 minutes. Stir once after 2 minutes of cooking.
4. Divide into 2 bowls and serve.

50. TOFU SCRAMBLE

Prep. time: 5 min | Cooking time: 10 min per crepe | Servings: 2

INGREDIENTS:

NUTRITIONAL VALUES PER SERVING: 1 CREPE (without toppings)	
Calories	100
Fat	6 g
Carbohydrates	4 g
Fiber	1 g
Protein	9 g
Sodium	208 mg
Potassium	232 mg
Phosphorus	183 mg

- ½ block extra-firm tofu, pressed of extra moisture, crumbled
- 1 tablespoon nutritional yeast
- ⅛ teaspoon pepper
- ½ tablespoon oil
- ⅛ teaspoon garlic salt
- ⅛ teaspoon turmeric powder

DIRECTIONS:

1. Pour oil into a skillet and heat it over medium heat. Once oil is hot, add turmeric powder and cook for 2-3 seconds.
2. Add tofu, pepper, and garlic salt and mix well. Heat thoroughly.
3. Add nutritional yeast and mix well. Cook for 2-3 minutes.
4. Divide into 2 plates and serve.

51. BERRY BAKED OATMEAL

Prep. time: 10 min | Cooking time: 30-40 min | Servings: 4

INGREDIENTS:

- ¼ cup chopped pecans, toasted
- 1 cup old fashioned rolled oats
- ¾ teaspoon ground cinnamon
- ⅛ teaspoon sea salt
- 2 tablespoons maple syrup
- ½ tablespoon butter
- ½ cup fresh or frozen blueberries
- ½ teaspoon baking powder
- ¼ teaspoon ground ginger
- 1 cup milk
- 1 small egg
- ½ teaspoon vanilla extract

NUTRITIONAL VALUES PER SERVING	
Calories	229
Fat	10 g
Carbohydrates	28 g
Fiber	4 g
Protein	6 g
Sodium	171 mg
Potassium	232 mg
Phosphorus	181 mg

DIRECTIONS:

1. Preheat your oven to 375°F. You can place the raw pecans on a baking sheet and place it in the oven while preheating the oven, it will get toasted.
2. Grease a small, square baking dish of about 4-5 inches with some cooking spray.
3. Mix together oats, baking powder, salt, pecans, and spices in a bowl.
4. Whisk together milk, egg, maple syrup, vanilla, and ¼ tablespoon butter in another bowl and whisk well.
5. Scatter half the berries in the baking dish. Spread oat mixture over the berries.
6. Spoon the milk mixture over the oat layer. Sprinkle the rest of the berries on top.
7. Place the baking dish in the oven and set the timer for about 30-40 minutes or until golden brown on top. Cool for about 5-8 minutes. Melt the remaining butter and drizzle on top.

52. BUCKWHEAT GROATS STRAWBERRY PORRIDGE

NUTRITIONAL VALUES PER SERVING	
Calories	124
Fat	2.1 g
Carbohydrates	24.8 g
Fiber	4 g
Protein	2.7 g
Sodium	455.5 mg
Potassium	20 mg
Phosphorus	0 mg

Prep. time: 5 min | Cooking time: 10 min | Servings: 1

INGREDIENTS:

- ¼ cup buckwheat groats
- 1 ¼ cups water
- A tiny pinch salt
- 1 teaspoon maple syrup or honey
- 1 stick cinnamon
- ½ cup unsweetened almond milk
- ½ cup chopped strawberries

DIRECTIONS:

1. Add water and cinnamon into a nonstick pan. Place the pan over medium heat.
2. When water starts boiling, stir in buckwheat and cook until tender.
3. Turn off the heat and pour into a bowl. Allow it to cool to room temperature.
4. Stir in honey and almond milk. Place strawberries on top and serve.

53. BLUEBERRY MUFFINS

Prep. time: 10 min | Cooking time: 30 min | Servings: 6
INGREDIENTS:

- ¼ cup unsalted butter
- 1 egg
- 1 cup all-purpose flour
- ¼ teaspoon salt
- 10 tablespoons sugar
- 1 teaspoon sugar for topping
- 1 cup 1% milk
- 1 teaspoon baking powder
- 1 ¼ cups fresh blueberries

NUTRITIONAL VALUES PER SERVING: 1 MUFFIN	
Calories	275
Fat	9 g
Carbohydrates	44 g
Fiber	1.3 g
Protein	5 g
Sodium	210 mg
Potassium	121 mg
Phosphorus	100 mg

DIRECTIONS:

1. While you are making the batter, preheat your oven to 375°F. Grease a 6 count muffin cup with cooking spray.
2. You can place disposable liners as well. This is optional.
3. Add butter and 10 tablespoons sugar into a mixing bowl and beat with an electric hand mixer on low speed until smooth and creamy.
4. Add egg and beat until well combined.
5. Sift together flour, salt, and baking powder in another bowl and stir. Add into the bowl of butter mixture a little at a time, alternating with a little milk each time.
6. Mash ¼ cup blueberries in a bowl. Add into the batter and mix using your hands.
7. Add the rest of the blueberries and mix using your hands.
8. Divide the batter among the muffin cups. Sprinkle 1 teaspoon sugar on top of the batter in the muffin cups.
9. Place the muffin pan in the oven and set the timer for about 25-30 minutes.
10. Remove the muffin pan from the oven and cool for 35-40 minutes and serve.

54. BREAKFAST BURRITO

Prep. time: 5 min | Cooking time: 3-10 min | Servings: 1
INGREDIENTS:

- 2 eggs
- ⅛ teaspoon ground cumin
- 1 flour tortilla, burrito size
- ¼ teaspoon hot pepper sauce
- 1 ½ tablespoon Ortega green chilies, sliced

NUTRITIONAL VALUES PER SERVING	
Calories	366
Fat	18 g
Carbohydrates	33 g
Fiber	2.5 g
Protein	18 g
Sodium	594 mg
Potassium	245 mg
Phosphorus	300 mg

DIRECTIONS:

1. Crack eggs into a bowl. Add hot sauce, green chilies, and cumin and whisk well.
2. Place a nonstick pan over medium heat. Spray the pan with cooking spray.
3. When the pan is hot, add the egg mixture and scramble the eggs. Cook until the eggs are done.
4. Warm the tortillas following the directions on the package.
5. Place the scrambled egg on the tortilla. Wrap like a burrito and serve.

55. VEGAN BUCKWHEAT BLUEBERRY MUFFINS

Prep. time: 10 min | Cooking time: 25 min | Servings: 6

INGREDIENTS:

- ½ cup + ⅛ cup almond milk
- ½ cup almond flour
- 11 tablespoons buckwheat flour
- ½ teaspoon baking powder
- ¼ teaspoon baking soda
- ¼ teaspoon ground cinnamon
- 2 tablespoons unrefined cane sugar or coconut sugar
- 2 tablespoons natural peanut butter or almond butter
- 1 teaspoon vanilla extract
- ½ teaspoon apple cider vinegar
- 1 ½ tablespoons melted coconut oil
- ¾ cup blueberries

NUTRITIONAL VALUES PER SERVING	
Calories	208
Fat	12 g
Carbohydrates	24 g
Fiber	3 g
Protein	5 g
Sodium	161 mg
Potassium	128 mg
Phosphorus	121 mg

DIRECTIONS:

1. While you are making the batter, preheat your oven to 350°F. Grease a 6 count muffin cup with cooking spray and place disposable liners as well (optional).
2. Combine almond milk and vinegar in a bowl to make buttermilk. Let it rest for 10 minutes.
3. Mix together buckwheat flour, baking soda, baking powder, almond flour, sugar, and cinnamon in a mixing bowl.
4. Whisk together peanut butter, vanilla, and coconut oil in another bowl. Pour the buttermilk and whisk until smooth. Pour the buttermilk mixture into the bowl of flour mixture. Mix until smooth.
5. Add most of the blueberries and fold gently.
6. Divide the batter among the muffin cups. Sprinkle remaining blueberries on top of the batter in the muffin cups. Press lightly to stick the berries but they should not sink in the batter.
7. Place the muffin pan in the oven and set the timer for about 25-30 minutes.
8. To check if the muffins are done, insert a toothpick in the center of the muffin. Pull the toothpick out. Check the toothpick to see if you can find any particles stuck on it. If you find any particles, you need to bake for some more time, maybe 5 minutes. If you do not see any particles stuck on the toothpick, the muffins are done and it is time to take the muffin pan out of the oven.
9. Let the muffins cool for a few minutes before taking them out of the pan. Serve them warm.

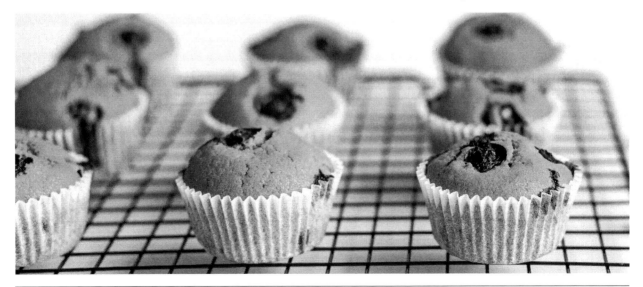

56. SOUTHWEST BREAKFAST TACOS

Prep. time: 20 min | Cooking time: 5 min | Servings: 1

INGREDIENTS:

- 2 taco shells (preferably use La Tiara)
- ¼ teaspoon Mrs. Dash taco seasoning
- 1 tablespoon diced red bell pepper
- 1 tablespoon fresh corn kernels
- 1 large egg
- 2 tablespoons shredded cheddar cheese
- A pinch salt (only to be added if taco shells do not contain salt)
- 1 tablespoon diced tomatoes
- 1 teaspoon unsalted butter
- 2 tablespoons chopped cilantro

NUTRITIONAL VALUES PER SERVING: 2 TACOS	
Calories	306
Fat	20 g
Carbohydrates	21 g
Fiber	2 g
Protein	12 g
Sodium	239 mg
Potassium	212 mg
Phosphorus	227 mg

DIRECTIONS:

1. Warm the taco shells following the directions on the package.
2. Meanwhile, whisk together egg, salt, and taco seasoning in a bowl.
3. Add corn, bell pepper, and tomatoes and stir.
4. Place a pan over medium heat. Add butter. When butter melts, add egg mixture and cook until eggs are soft and creamy, stirring occasionally. Turn off the heat but keep stirring for about a minute.
5. Divide the egg mixture among the taco shells. Place a tablespoon of cheese in each taco. Garnish with cilantro and serve.

57. EGG SALAD ENGLISH MUFFIN BREAKFAST SANDWICH

Prep. time: 15 min | Cooking time: 10 min per crepe | Servings: 2

INGREDIENTS:

- 6 hard boiled eggs, peeled, discard yolks
- ½ teaspoon minced dill
- 4 tablespoons homemade kidney-friendly mayonnaise
- 12 cucumber slices
- 2 English muffins, split, toasted

NUTRITIONAL VALUES PER SERVING: 2 OPEN-FACED SANDWICHES	
Calories	387
Fat	23.2 g
Carbohydrates	28.7 g
Fiber	0.3 g
Protein	16 g
Sodium	370.6 mg
Potassium	236.1 mg
Phosphorus	32.8 mg

DIRECTIONS:

1. Finely chop the whites and add into a bowl. Add dill and mayonnaise and stir.
2. Place 3 cucumber slices on each muffin half. Divide the egg salad over the muffin halves and serve.

58. POLENTA AND EGG BREAKFAST CUPS

Prep. time: 10-12 min | Cooking time: 15-18 min | Servings: 2

INGREDIENTS:

- 3 ounces tubed polenta, cut into 2 equal portions
- 2 large eggs
- A pinch kosher salt
- ⅛ cup diced small Roma tomatoes
- 1 ounce shredded cheddar cheese, divided
- 2 teaspoons unsalted butter
- 1 tablespoon Mexican crema or sour cream
- 1 teaspoon Mrs. Dash taco seasoning
- ⅛ cup diced red bell pepper
- ⅛ cup thinly sliced green onion
- 1 tablespoon chopped cilantro

NUTRITIONAL VALUES PER SERVING: 1 CREPE (without toppings)	
Calories	216
Fat	5 g
Carbohydrates	9 g
Fiber	1 g
Protein	11 g
Sodium	347 mg
Potassium	172 mg
Phosphorus	195 mg

DIRECTIONS:

1. Set your oven to broil mode and preheat the oven to highest heat.
2. Take 2 ramekins and grease it with some cooking spray. Crumble a piece of polenta in each ramekin.
3. Add a teaspoon of butter into each ramekin and place in the oven. Broil until light brown.
4. Meanwhile, crack eggs into a bowl. Add salt and taco seasoning and whisk well.
5. Stir in onion, tomato, and red bell pepper.
6. Scatter a tablespoon of cheese in each ramekin. Distribute the vegetable mixture among the ramekins. Place the ramekins in the oven and cook until the eggs are cooked.
7. Sprinkle remaining cheese on top. Let them rest for 2-3 minutes.
8. Garnish with cilantro and crema and serve.

59. SPICED EGGNOG

Prep. time: 2-3 min | Cooking time: 0 min | Servings: 3

INGREDIENTS:

- 1 cup half and half
- 2 tablespoons sugar
- ¼ teaspoon pumpkin pie spice
- 3 tablespoons whipped cream
- 6 tablespoons low cholesterol egg product
- 1 teaspoon rum extract
- ⅛ teaspoon ground nutmeg

NUTRITIONAL VALUES PER SERVING	
Calories	162
Fat	10 g
Carbohydrates	13 g
Fiber	0 g
Protein	5 g
Sodium	78 mg
Potassium	149 mg
Phosphorus	83 mg

DIRECTIONS:

1. Chill the blender jar in the freezer for about 20 minutes before preparing the eggnog.
2. Place sugar, pumpkin pie spice, egg product, rum extract, and nutmeg in the chilled blender and blend until smooth.
3. Divide into 3 small glasses. Place a tablespoon of whipped topping on top of each glass. Sprinkle nutmeg and serve.

60. MINI FRITTATAS

Prep. time: 15 min | Cooking time: 30-40 min | Servings: 4

INGREDIENTS:

- ½ pound frozen hash brown potatoes
- 1 tablespoon diced green bell pepper
- 1 tablespoon diced red bell pepper
- 1 ounce cooked lean ham
- 1 tablespoon minced onion
- ½ tablespoon 1% low fat milk
- ¼ cup shredded low-fat cheddar cheese
- A pinch black pepper
- 2 large eggs

NUTRITIONAL VALUES PER SERVING: 1 FRITTATA	
Calories	112
Fat	4 g
Carbohydrates	11 g
Fiber	1 g
Protein	8 g
Sodium	115 mg
Potassium	162 mg
Phosphorus	134 mg

DIRECTIONS:

1. Place hash browns potatoes in a bowl. Pour enough water to cover the hash browns. Drain off after 4 hours. Rinse well. Hold the hash browns between your palms and squeeze out as much water as possible. This is to be done only if low potassium is required.
2. Preheat your oven to 375°F.
3. Grease 4 ramekins or muffin cups with some cooking spray. Divide the hash browns among the cups and press it well onto the bottom of the cups.
4. Spray some cooking spray over the hash browns. Place the muffin cups in the oven and set the timer for 15 minutes.
5. Take out the muffin cups from the oven and lower the temperature of your oven to 350°F.
6. Whisk eggs and milk in a bowl. Add pepper, ham, onion, and bell pepper and mix well.
7. Take a spoon and press the hash browns well onto the bottom of the cups.
8. Divide the vegetable mixture equally among the muffin cups. Place the cups back in the oven and bake until golden brown on top and the eggs are set. Cool for 5 minutes.

61. QUINOA PORRIDGE

Prep. time: 10 min | Cooking time: 15 min | Servings: 2

INGREDIENTS:

- ½ cup Quinoa rinsed and drained
- 1 cup of fresh fruits
- 2 tablespoons chopped nuts
- 1 tablespoon maple syrup
- 1 cup water

NUTRITIONAL VALUES PER SERVING: ½ CUP (without fruits)	
Calories	200
Calcium	18 g
Protein	35 g
Sodium	75 mg
Potassium	31 mg
Phosphorus	80 mg

DIRECTIONS:

1. Add the quinoa and water in a medium saucepan
2. Bring it to a boil and then let it simmer with the lid on for 10-15 min or until the quinoa is soft
3. Once cooked, remove from heat and let it sit on the counter for 10 minutes. Split into two bowls
4. Top it off with the fresh fruits, chopped nuts and maple syrup. Stir thoroughly before serving.

CHAPTER 8
Lunch Recipes

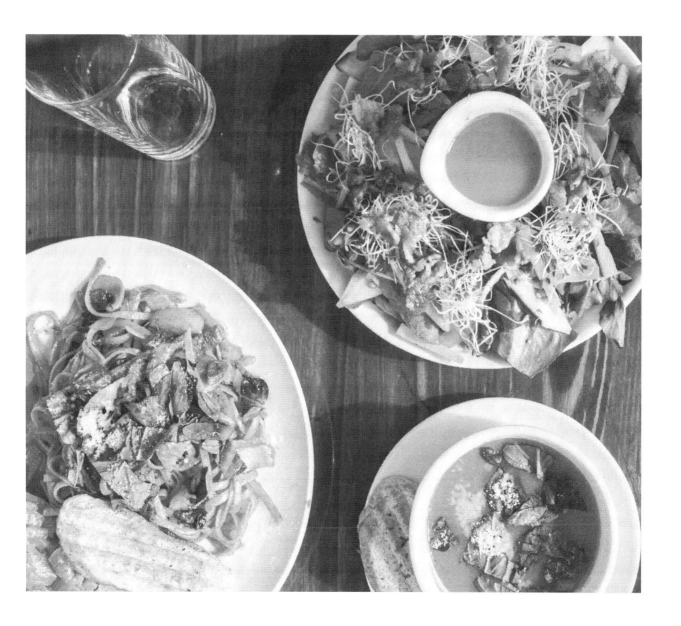

62. GARDEN SALAD

Prep. time: 10 min | Cooking time: 0 min | Servings: 1

INGREDIENTS:

- ¾ cup Romaine lettuce
- ¼ small tomato, diced
- ¼ cucumber, diced
- ½ stalk celery, diced
- 1 cup iceberg lettuce
- 2 baby carrots, shredded
- ¼ red onion, diced
- ½ teaspoon olive oil
- 1 teaspoon vinegar

NUTRITIONAL VALUES PER SERVING	
Calories	24
Fat	0.2 g
Carbohydrates	5.4 g
Protein	1.1 g
Sodium	18.6 mg
Potassium	232.8 mg
Phosphorus	31.4 mg

DIRECTIONS:

Place all the vegetables in a bowl. Add oil and vinegar and toss well. Serve

63. BOW-TIE PASTA SALAD

Prep. time: 5 min | Cooking time: 0 min + chilling time | Servings: 2

INGREDIENTS:

- 1 cup cooked bow tie pasta
- 1 tablespoon chopped green bell pepper
- 1 tablespoon minced onion
- ⅓ cup low fat mayonnaise
- ½ tablespoon lemon juice
- ¼ teaspoon sugar
- ⅛ cup chopped celery
- 1 tablespoon shredded carrot
- A pinch pepper

NUTRITIONAL VALUES PER SERVING	
Calories	188
Fat	9.4 g
Carbohydrates	22.2 g
Protein	3.4 g
Sodium	339.6 mg
Potassium	84.6 mg
Phosphorus	42.8 mg

DIRECTIONS:

1. Combine mayonnaise, pepper, sugar, and lemon juice in a bowl.
2. Add vegetables and pasta and mix well.
3. Chill and serve.

64. APPLE CRANBERRY WALNUT SALAD

Prep. time: 15 min | Cooking time: 0 min + chilling time | Servings: 5-6

INGREDIENTS:

- 1 cup halved red seedless grapes
- 3 ounces pomegranate infused Ocean Spray dried cranberries
- 3 ½ medium Gala apples, cored, chopped into bite size pieces
- ⅔ cup walnut halves, chopped
- 2 stalks celery, cut into ¼ inch pieces
- 4 ounces Maple Grove Farms of Vermont Fat-free cranberry balsamic dressing

NUTRITIONAL VALUES PER SERVING: ½ CUP	
Calories	94
Fat	3.5 g
Carbohydrates	15.7 g
Protein	1 g
Sodium	60.7 mg
Potassium	102.6 mg
Phosphorus	26.2 mg

DIRECTIONS:

1. Combine all the fruits, walnuts, and celery in a bowl.
2. Pour dressing on top. Toss well and serve.

65. COUSCOUS SALAD WITH TANGY DRESSING

Prep. time: 20 min | Cooking time: 30 min + chilling time | Servings: 6-7

INGREDIENTS:

- ½ tablespoon minced garlic
- ½ teaspoon ground allspice
- Juice of a lemon
- ¼ cup frozen corn
- ¼ cup chopped red bell pepper
- ¼ cup chopped yellow bell pepper
- 1 ½ large cucumbers, peeled, cubed
- ½ teaspoon dried oregano
- ½ tablespoon olive oil
- ½ cup whole sugar snap peas
- ¼ cup chopped carrots
- ½ cup dry couscous

NUTRITIONAL VALUES PER SERVING: ½ CUP	
Calories	151
Fat	2.5 g
Carbohydrates	28.7 g
Protein	4.9 g
Sodium	14.3 mg
Potassium	353.9 mg
Phosphorus	94 mg

DIRECTIONS:

1. Cook the couscous following the directions on the package.
2. Cool completely and chill for an hour or so.
3. Combine couscous and vegetables in a bowl and toss well.
4. To make dressing: Combine lemon juice, oil, garlic, and spices in a bowl. Pour the dressing over the salad.
5. Toss well. Cover and chill for a few hours.

66. LEMON ORZO SPRING SALAD

Prep. time: 5-10 min | Cooking time: 10 min per crepe | Servings: 2

INGREDIENTS:

- ¼ cup + ⅛ cup orzo pasta
- ⅛ cup diced green bell pepper
- ⅛ cup diced red bell pepper
- ⅛ cup diced yellow bell pepper
- ¼ cup diced onion
- 3 tablespoons olive oil
- ½ teaspoon lemon zest
- ¼ teaspoon dried oregano
- 1 tablespoon chopped fresh rosemary
- 1 cup cubed zucchini
- 1 ½ tablespoons fresh lemon juice
- 1 ½ tablespoons grated parmesan cheese
- ¼ teaspoon ground black pepper
- ⅛ teaspoon red pepper flakes

NUTRITIONAL VALUES PER SERVING: 1½ CUPS	
Calories	330
Fat	22 g
Carbohydrates	28 g
Protein	6 g
Sodium	79 mg
Potassium	376 mg
Phosphorus	134 mg

DIRECTIONS:

1. Follow the directions on the package of pasta and cook the pasta. Drain in a colander. Do not rinse the orzo after cooking.
2. Place a pan over medium heat with a tablespoon of oil. When oil is hot, add onion, bell peppers, and zucchini and cook until onion turns soft. Turn off the heat.
3. Combine lemon juice, 2 tablespoon oil, rosemary, lemon zest, cheese, pepper, red pepper flakes, and oregano in a bowl.
4. Add the cooked vegetables and orzo and fold gently. Serve.

67. CRUNCHY QUINOA SALAD

Prep. time: 15 min | Cooking time: 10-12 min | Servings: 4

INGREDIENTS:

- ½ cup quinoa, rinsed well
- 1 cup water
- 2-3 cherry tomatoes, halved
- 1 ½ green onions, chopped
- ¼ cup chopped flat-leaf parsley
- ½ tablespoon grated lemon zest
- ⅛ cup grated parmesan cheese
- 1 cup water
- ¼ cup peeled, diced cucumber
- ⅛ cup chopped fresh mint
- 1 tablespoon fresh lemon juice
- 2 tablespoons olive oil
- ¼ head Boston or Bibb lettuce leaves, separated into cups

NUTRITIONAL VALUES PER SERVING: 2 LETTUCE CUPS	
Calories	158
Fat	9 g
Carbohydrates	16 g
Protein	5 g
Sodium	46 mg
Potassium	237 mg
Phosphorus	129 mg

DIRECTIONS:

1. Place a pan over medium-high heat. Add quinoa and stir-fry for a couple of minutes until toasted.
2. Pour water and let the mixture come to a boil.
3. Lower the heat and cook covered until dry. Turn off the heat. Let it sit covered for 5 minutes.
4. Take a fork and fluff the quinoa. Spread on a plate to cool completely.
5. Add quinoa, cucumber, tomatoes, onion, lemon juice, oil, lemon zest, and herbs into a bowl and toss well.
6. Arrange the lettuce cups on a large serving platter. Place ¼ cup salad in each lettuce cup.
7. Garnish with parmesan cheese and serve.

68. CABBAGE ONION SWEET PEPPER MEDLEY

Prep. time: 10 min | Cooking time: 8-10 min | Servings: 2

INGREDIENTS:

- ¼ cup sliced green bell pepper
- ¼ cup sliced red bell pepper
- ¼ cup sliced yellow bell pepper
- 1 cup shredded cabbage
- ¼ cup sliced onion
- ½ tablespoon canola oil
- ¾ teaspoon Dijon mustard
- 1 ½ tablespoons white vinegar
- ¾ teaspoon brown sugar
- ¾ teaspoon pepper

NUTRITIONAL VALUES PER SERVING	
Calories	70
Fat	4 g
Carbohydrates	8 g
Protein	1 g
Sodium	52 mg
Potassium	208 mg
Phosphorus	29 mg

DIRECTIONS:

1. The bell peppers should be cut into 2 inch strips.
2. Place bell peppers, cabbage, and onion in a pan and cook for a few minutes until slightly tender and crunchy.
3. Whisk together oil, mustard, vinegar, brown sugar, and pepper in a small bowl.
4. Pour the mixture into the pan and mix well. Once the cabbage is tender, turn off the heat.
5. Divide into 2 plates and serve.

69. CURRIED TOFU SALAD

Prep. time: 10 min | Cooking time: 0 min | Servings: 2

INGREDIENTS:

- 3.5 ounces firm tofu, crumbled
- ½ medium carrot, grated
- 1 ½ tablespoons vegan mayonnaise
- Freshly ground pepper to taste
- 1 ½ scallions, sliced
- 3 tablespoons raisins
- 1 ½ tablespoons chopped walnuts
- ¾ tablespoon curry powder
- A tiny pinch salt

NUTRITIONAL VALUES PER SERVING: ¾ CUP	
Calories	168
Fat	9 g
Carbohydrates	17 g
Protein	8 g
Sodium	144 mg
Potassium	310 mg
Phosphorus	128 mg

DIRECTIONS:

1. Combine all the ingredients in a bowl and stir until well combined.
2. Divide into 2 bowls and serve.

70. APPLE RICE SALAD

Prep. time: 10 min | Cooking time: 0 min | Servings: 2

INGREDIENTS:

DRESSING:
- 1 tablespoon balsamic vinegar
- 1 teaspoon honey
- ½ tablespoon finely shredded orange zest
- ½ tablespoon olive oil
- 1 teaspoon brown or Dijon mustard
- ⅛ teaspoon garlic powder

SALAD:
- 1 cup cooked white rice, chilled
- ½ cup thinly sliced celery
- 1 medium apple, cored, chopped
- 1 tablespoons shelled, unsalted sunflower seeds

NUTRITIONAL VALUES PER SERVING: ¾ CUP	
Calories	238
Fat	6 g
Carbohydrates	42 g
Protein	4 g
Sodium	227 mg
Potassium	238 mg
Phosphorus	82 mg

DIRECTIONS:

1. Whisk together all the dressing ingredients in a bowl.
2. Add salad ingredients in another bowl. Toss well.
3. Pour dressing over the salad. Toss well.
4. Serve at room temperature or chill and serve later.

71. ASIAN PEAR SALAD

Prep. time: 10 min | Cooking time: 5 min | Servings: 2

INGREDIENTS:

- ¼ cup water
- ¼ cup sugar
- ¼ cup chopped walnuts
- 2 Asian pears, peeled, cored, diced
- ¼ cup pomegranate arils
- 3 cups torn lettuces leaves
- 1 ounce stilton or blue cheese
- 1 teaspoon olive oil
- 1 teaspoon vinegar

NUTRITIONAL VALUES PER SERVING	
Calories	301
Fat	2.3 g
Carbohydrates	41 g
Protein	6 g
Sodium	206 mg
Potassium	297 mg
Phosphorus	127 mg

DIRECTIONS:

1. Combine sugar and water in a nonstick pan. Place the pan over medium-low heat and cook until you get syrup.
2. Add walnuts and stir. Turn off the heat.
3. Line a plate with parchment paper. Spread the walnuts on the plate. Keep it aside until it cools completely.
4. Combine lettuce, pears, cheese, pomegranate, oil, and vinegar in a bowl.
5. Toss well and divide into 2 plates. Garnish with sugar coated walnuts on top and serve

72. BERRY WILD RICE SALAD

Prep. time: 4 min | Cooking time: 20 min | Servings: 4

INGREDIENTS:

- 1 cup water
- 1 cup uncooked wild rice
- ½ cup collard greens, slightly steamed
- ⅛ cup blueberries
- 1 ¼ cups mixed berries of your choice (apart from blueberries)
- ¼ cup chopped onion

DRESSING:
- 1 tablespoon lemon juice
- ½ tablespoon olive oil
- ⅛ cup chopped fresh mint
- ¼ cup fat-free or low-fat sour cream

NUTRITIONAL VALUES PER SERVING	
Calories	133
Fat	4 g
Carbohydrates	25 g
Protein	4 g
Sodium	26 mg
Potassium	159 mg
Phosphorus	111 mg

DIRECTIONS:

1. Combine rice and water in a saucepan. Place the saucepan over high heat.
2. When water starts boiling, lower the heat and cover with a lid. Simmer until nearly dry.
3. Turn off the heat and transfer the wild rice into a bowl. Add collard greens, blueberries, mixed berries, and onion and toss well.
4. Blend together mint, oil, and lemon juice in a blender until smooth.
5. Pour into a bowl. Add sour cream and whisk until well incorporated.
6. Pour dressing over the salad. Toss well.
7. Divide into 4 equal portions and serve at room temperature or chilled.

73. COLD SESAME NOODLE SALAD

Prep. time: 20 min | Cooking time: 20 min + chilling time | Servings: 6

INGREDIENTS:

DRESSING:
- ¼ cup finely grated onion
- 4-5 tablespoons fresh lemon juice
- 4 tablespoons sesame oil
- 2 teaspoons rice vinegar
- 2 medium pears, peeled, cored, finely grated (1 cup is required)
- 4 tablespoons low-sodium soy sauce
- 2 tablespoons sesame seeds

SALAD:
- 2 cups soybean sprouts
- 10 ounces dried buckwheat noodles
- 8 cups shredded lettuce leaves
- 2 medium carrots, julienne cut
- 2 small cucumbers, julienne cut
- 1 tablespoon black sesame seeds (optional)
- 1 tablespoon white sesame seeds

NUTRITIONAL VALUES PER SERVING: ¾ CUP	
Calories	392
Fat	14.9 g
Carbohydrates	57.6 g
Protein	15.5 g
Sodium	477.1 mg
Potassium	580.4 mg
Phosphorus	191.8 mg

DIRECTIONS:

1. Combine all the dressing ingredients in a bowl. Cover the bowl and chill until ready to use. You can also blend the dressing ingredients in a blender if you do not want to grate the onion and pears. You can chop them into pieces and blend it along with other ingredients.
2. Cook the sprouts in a pot of boiling water until it still has some crunch.
3. Remove the sprouts with a slotted spoon and place on a strainer or colander.
4. Add carrots into the boiling water and remove them with a slotted spoon and place it on the strainer along with sprouts. After a couple of minutes, transfer into a bowl.
5. Drop the noodles into the boiling water and cook until al dente. Finally, drain off the noodles in the strainer and rinse under cold running water. Drain well for a few minutes in the strainer and transfer it into the bowl of sprouts. Add cucumber into the bowl. Pour dressing and stir gently.
6. Cover the bowl and chill for a few hours before serving.
7. If you want to lower the potassium levels to 435 mg for every serving, use apple instead of pear, 1 cup bell pepper slices instead of carrot and use mung bean sprouts instead of soybean sprouts. Do not garnish with sesame seeds.

74. PIMENTO CREAM CHEESE SANDWICHES

NUTRITIONAL VALUES PER SERVING: 4 TABLESPOONS SPREAD WITH 4 SLICES	
Calories	304
Fat	16 g
Carbohydrates	32 g
Protein	8 g
Sodium	411 mg
Potassium	137 mg
Phosphorus	101 mg

Prep. time: 5 min | Cooking time: 0 min | Servings: 4

INGREDIENTS:

- 1 cup whipped cream cheese
- 1 teaspoon sugar
- 8 slices white bread
- 2 tablespoons chopped canned pimento
- ¼ teaspoon pepper

DIRECTIONS:

1. Mix together pimento, cream cheese, pepper, and sugar in a bowl.
2. Spread 4 tablespoons mixture in between 2 slices of bread. Cut into desired shape and serve.

75. TURKEY WALDORF SALAD

Prep. time: 10 min | Cooking time: 0 min | Servings: 3

INGREDIENTS:

- 6 ounces unsalted turkey breast, cooked, cubed
- ½ cup sliced celery
- 1 ½ medium apples, cored, diced
- ¼ cup diced onion
- 1 tablespoon apple juice
- 2 tablespoons mayonnaise— refer to the Vegetarian Reuben sandwich for the recipe

NUTRITIONAL VALUES PER SERVING: ½ CUP	
Calories	200
Fat	11 g
Carbohydrates	8 g
Protein	296 g
Sodium	128 mg
Potassium	296 mg
Phosphorus	136 mg

DIRECTIONS:

1. Add apple, turkey, onion, and celery into a bowl and toss well. Stir in mayonnaise and apple juice.
2. Cover the bowl and chill until use.

76. MINESTRONE SOUP

Prep. time: 10 min | Cooking time: 20 min | Servings: 3-4

INGREDIENTS:

- ½ can (from a 14 ounce can) unsalted diced tomatoes
- 2 cups low-fat, low-sodium chicken broth
- ½ teaspoon dried basil
- ½ teaspoon dried oregano
- ¼ cup chopped zucchini
- 1 large stalk celery, chopped
- ½ large carrot, shredded
- 1 small onion, chopped
- 1 clove garlic, minced
- ¾ cup fresh green snap beans (½ inch pieces)
- 1 tablespoon olive oil
- ¾ cup dry elbow macaroni

NUTRITIONAL VALUES PER SERVING: 1 CUP	
Calories	144
Fat	4.3 g
Carbohydrates	21.9 g
Protein	5.9 g
Sodium	55.1 mg
Potassium	355.2 mg
Phosphorus	97.8 mg

DIRECTIONS:

1. Pour oil into a soup pot and let it heat over medium heat. Once oil is hot, add onion and cook until it turns pink.
2. Stir in garlic and fresh vegetables and mix well. Cook until the vegetables are slightly tender.
3. Stir in tomatoes, broth, oregano, basil, and pepper. Lower the heat and let it cook until the vegetables are tender.
4. Meanwhile, cook macaroni following the directions on the package.
5. Add macaroni into the pot and mix well.
6. Serve hot.

77. CURRIED CARROT SOUP

Prep. time: 10 min | Cooking time: 20 min | Servings: 3

INGREDIENTS:

- 2 tablespoons avocado oil
- ¾ pound baby carrots (Substituting half the carrots with cauliflower will reduce the potassium)
- ¾ tablespoon curry powder
- 1 ½ cups low sodium vegetable broth (Using unsalted broth will bring down the sodium levels)
- ⅛ teaspoon sea salt
- ½ medium onion, diced
- ¾ inch fresh ginger, minced
- ¼ teaspoon red pepper flakes
- ½ can (from a 15 ounces can) coconut milk (Using rice milk instead of coconut milk will bring down the potassium)
- ⅛ teaspoon black pepper
- Lemon juice to taste
- 1 ½ tablespoons finely chopped chives

NUTRITIONAL VALUES PER SERVING: 1 CUP	
Calories	286
Fat	25 g
Carbohydrates	15.09 g
Protein	3 g
Sodium	256.1 mg
Potassium	578 mg
Phosphorus	156.5 mg

DIRECTIONS:

1. Pour oil into a pot and place the pot over medium heat. When oil is hot, add onion and cook until tender. Stir in ginger and carrots and cook for about 3-4 minutes, stirring occasionally.
2. Stir in red pepper flakes and curry powder. Stir for a few seconds until you get a nice aroma, making sure not to burn the spices.
3. Retain about 2 tablespoons of the coconut milk and pour the rest into the pot. Also pour in the broth and stir. When it begins to boil, reduce the heat, cover, and cook until the carrots are cooked. Blend the soup with an immersion blender until smooth. Add salt and pepper and stir.
4. Ladle into soup bowls and serve.

78. GROUND BEEF SOUP

Prep. time: 10 min | Cooking time: 25-30 min | Servings: 3

INGREDIENTS:

- ½ pound lean ground beef
- 1 teaspoon Mrs. Dash lemon pepper seasoning blend
- ½ cup low-sodium beef broth
- 3 tablespoons uncooked white rice
- ½ tablespoon sour cream
- ¼ cup chopped onion
- ½ teaspoon Kitchen bouquet seasoning and browning sauce
- 1 cup water
- 1 ½ cups frozen mixed vegetables (green beans, carrots, peas, and corn)

NUTRITIONAL VALUES PER SERVING: 1¼ CUPS	
Calories	222
Fat	8 g
Carbohydrates	19 g
Protein	20 g
Sodium	170 mg
Potassium	448 mg
Phosphorus	210 mg

DIRECTIONS:

1. Place a saucepan over medium heat. Add meat and onion and cook until meat is brown. Discard the excess fat from the saucepan.
2. Stir in browning sauce, Mrs. Dash seasoning, rice, broth, vegetables, and water.
3. When water starts boiling, lower the heat to medium-low and cook covered for about 20 minutes until vegetables are cooked. Add sour cream and stir. Ladle into a soup bowl.

79. BEAN SOUP

Prep. time: 5 min | Cooking time: 15 min | Servings: 3

INGREDIENTS:

- ½ can (from a 16 ounces can) fat-free, unsalted chicken broth
- ½ can (from a 14.4 ounce can) unsalted diced tomatoes
- ½ can (from a 14.4 ounce can) unsalted corn, drained, rinsed
- ½ can (from a 14.4 ounce can) fat-free refried beans
- ½ can (from a 14.4 ounce can) unsalted black beans, drained, rinsed

NUTRITIONAL VALUES PER SERVING: 1¼ CUP	
Calories	214
Fat	2 g
Carbohydrates	39 g
Protein	13 g
Sodium	296 mg
Potassium	762 mg
Phosphorus	236 mg

DIRECTIONS:

1. Add broth, beans, tomatoes, corn, and refried beans into a saucepan and stir.
2. Place the saucepan over medium heat and stir often until refried beans are well-blended with the broth. Heat thoroughly. Ladle into soup bowls and serve.

80. BAKED POTATO SOUP

Prep. time: 5 min | Cooking time: 45 min | Servings: 3

INGREDIENTS:

- 1 large potato, peeled
- 2 cups skim-milk
- 3 tablespoons flour
- ¼ teaspoon pepper
- ¼ cup fat-free sour cream
- 2 ounces shredded low-fat Monterey Jack cheese

NUTRITIONAL VALUES PER SERVING: 1½ CUPS	
Calories	216
Fat	1 g
Carbohydrates	29 g
Protein	15 g
Sodium	272 mg
Potassium	594 mg
Phosphorus	326 mg

DIRECTIONS:

1. Set the temperature of your oven to 400°F. Place potato on a baking sheet and place it in the oven for about 25-30 minutes or until cooked through.
2. Mash the potato well. Whisk together milk and flour in a saucepan. Place the saucepan over medium heat and stir constantly, add potato and pepper.
3. Stir often until thick. Stir in cheese. Once cheese melts, turn off the heat.
4. Add sour cream and stir. Ladle into soup bowls and serve.

81. SPAGHETTI-BASIL FRITTATA

Prep. time: 5 min | Cooking time: 10 min | Servings: 2

INGREDIENTS:

- 3 tablespoons sliced green onion
- 1 ¼ cups cooked whole wheat spaghetti
- White of a large egg
- 2 large eggs
- ⅛ teaspoon black pepper
- 1 tablespoon chopped basil
- 3 tablespoons 1% low-fat milk
- 1 ounce mozzarella cheese, shredded
- 1 teaspoon olive oil

NUTRITIONAL VALUES PER SERVING: 2 WEDGES	
Calories	271
Fat	11 g
Carbohydrates	26 g
Protein	17 g
Sodium	208 mg
Potassium	212 mg
Phosphorus	279 mg

DIRECTIONS:

1. Pour oil into a small skillet and heat over medium heat. Place spaghetti and stir. Cook for a couple of minutes.
2. Add egg white, eggs, milk, and pepper into a bowl and whisk well.
3. Pour into the skillet, all over the spaghetti. Scatter green onion, cheese, and basil on top. Do not stir. Cover the skillet and cook until the eggs are set.
4. Turn off the heat. Loosen the frittata by sliding a spatula below it. Cut into 4 equal wedges and serve.

82. SPICY FRITTATA

Prep. time: 10 min | Cooking time: 10 min | Servings: 2

INGREDIENTS:

- 2 egg whites
- 1 large egg
- A pinch turmeric powder
- A pinch black pepper
- ¼ cup finely chopped onion
- 1 cup thinly sliced zucchini
- ½ small tomato, chopped
- ⅛ teaspoon salt
- ½ tablespoon chicken broth
- 2 small cloves garlic, minced
- 1 tablespoon canned chopped chilies
- 1 tablespoon chopped cilantro

NUTRITIONAL VALUES PER SERVING: 2 WEDGES	
Calories	87
Fat	3 g
Carbohydrates	7 g
Protein	8 g
Sodium	256 mg
Potassium	360 mg
Phosphorus	96 mg

DIRECTIONS:

1. Add egg whites, eggs, salt, pepper and turmeric into a bowl and whisk well.
2. Pour broth into a small skillet and place the skillet over medium heat.
3. Add garlic, onion, green chili, and zucchini and cook for 2-3 minutes.
4. Stir in tomato and cilantro. Cook for about a minute. Spread the vegetables all over the pan.
5. Drizzle the egg mixture all over the vegetables in the pan. Do not stir. Cover the skillet and cook until the eggs are set.
6. Turn off the heat. Loosen the frittata by sliding a spatula below it. Cut into 4 equal wedges and serve.

83. ALASKAN BAKED MACARONI AND CHEESE

Prep. time: 5 min | Cooking time: 30 min | Servings: 4

INGREDIENTS:

- 1 ½ cups elbow pasta
- 1 cup grated cheddar cheese
- ½ teaspoon mustard powder
- ½ tablespoon fresh tarragon or thyme, or ½ teaspoon dried
- 1 tablespoon flour
- 1 cup milk
- ½ teaspoon paprika
- 1 tablespoon unsalted butter
- Chopped almonds to garnish (optional)

NUTRITIONAL VALUES PER SERVING	
Calories	424
Fat	20 g
Carbohydrates	36 g
Protein	2 g
Sodium	479 mg
Potassium	237 mg
Phosphorus	428 mg

DIRECTIONS:

1. Add water into a pot and place over high heat. Add pasta and cook until al dente. Drain and place in a bowl.
2. Set the temperature of your oven to 350°F and preheat the oven.
3. Place a pan over medium heat. Add butter. Once butter melts, add flour and stir constantly until roux is formed.
4. Pour milk stirring constantly. Keep stirring until thick.
5. Add pasta and cheddar cheese and stir. Turn off the heat. Transfer the pasta into a baking dish.
6. Place the baking dish in the oven for 15 minutes. Sprinkle almonds on top. Continue baking for another 5-6 minutes.
7. Serve hot.

84. EGG FRIED RICE

Prep. time: 5 min | Cooking time: 3-4 min | Servings: 5

INGREDIENTS:

- 1 teaspoon dark sesame oil
- 1 egg white
- 1 egg
- ½ tablespoon canola oil
- ½ cup frozen peas, thawed
- 3 tablespoons chopped green onion
- ½ cup bean sprouts
- 2 cups, cooked rice cold
- ⅛ teaspoon pepper

NUTRITIONAL VALUES PER SERVING: ½ CUP	
Calories	137
Fat	4 g
Carbohydrates	21 g
Protein	5 g
Sodium	38 mg
Potassium	89 mg
Phosphorus	67 mg

DIRECTIONS:

1. Stir together sesame oil, egg white, and whole egg in a bowl.
2. Pour oil into a nonstick pan and heat over medium-high heat. When the oil is hot, add egg mixture and stir often until the eggs are cooked.
3. Stir in the green onion and bean sprouts. Cook for a couple of minutes, stirring often.
4. Add rice, peas, and pepper and mix well. Heat thoroughly.
5. Serve.

85. CRUNCHY CHICKEN WRAPS

Prep. time: 5 min | Cooking time: 0 min | Servings: 2

INGREDIENTS:

- ½ stalk celery, diced
- ¼ red bell pepper, diced
- ¼ teaspoon onion powder
- 4 ounces canned, low-sodium chicken
- ½ medium carrot, diced
- 2 tablespoons low-fat mayonnaise
- 1 lavash wrap

NUTRITIONAL VALUES PER SERVING: ½ WRAP	
Calories	260
Fat	9 g
Carbohydrates	27 g
Protein	17 g
Sodium	462 mg
Potassium	215 mg
Phosphorus	103 mg

DIRECTIONS:

1. Mix together onion powder and mayonnaise in a bowl and spread it over the wrap.
2. Scatter the vegetables and chicken on one half of the wrap. Roll it up and place it with its seam side down. Cut into 2 halves. Fix the halves with toothpicks and serve. To reduce the sodium levels, cook chicken at home without adding any salt.

86. CHILLED SUMMER SQUASH AND TURMERIC SOUP

Prep. time: 5 min | Cooking time: 30 min | Servings: 3

INGREDIENTS:

- 2 cups low-sodium vegetable broth
- 1 medium yellow squash, chopped into chunks
- ¼ cup frozen peas
- ¼ teaspoon kosher salt
- 1 teaspoon turmeric powder
- 1 medium zucchini, chopped
- into chunks
- ½ small onion, diced
- 1 tablespoon olive oil
- ¼ cup plain, nonfat Greek yogurt

NUTRITIONAL VALUES PER SERVING: 1 CUP	
Calories	100
Fat	5 g
Carbohydrates	10 g
Protein	4 g
Sodium	279 mg
Potassium	504 mg
Phosphorus	138 mg

DIRECTIONS:

1. Combine zucchini, onion, and squash in a saucepan. Add broth and cook until tender.
2. Add peas, salt, turmeric powder, and oil and cook until the peas are soft. Turn off the heat and let it cool completely.
3. Blend the mixture with an immersion blender until smooth.
4. Add Greek yogurt and stir. Chill for 6-8 hours and serve.

87. VEGETABLE PAELLA

Prep. time: 5 min | Cooking time: 30 min | Servings: 4

INGREDIENTS:

- 1 cup sliced asparagus
- ½ tablespoon olive oil
- 1 small zucchini, diced (about ⅔ cup)
- 1 ½ cups broccoli florets
- ½ cup diced green bell pepper
- ¼ cup diced onion
- ¼ teaspoon saffron
- ¼ teaspoon salt
- 1 cup uncooked rice, rinsed

NUTRITIONAL VALUES PER SERVING: 1¼ CUPS	
Calories	146
Fat	2 g
Carbohydrates	26 g
Protein	5 g
Sodium	150 mg
Potassium	5 mg
Phosphorus	89 mg

DIRECTIONS:

1. Cook rice following the directions on the package. Cook asparagus and broccoli in a pot of water until crisp as well as tender. Drain in a colander.
2. Pour oil into a skillet and heat it over medium heat. Add the vegetables and sauté until the vegetables are tender.
3. Add saffron and salt and mix well. Add rice and mix well. Cook for a couple of minutes or until well heated.

88. TUNA-SALAD SANDWICH

Prep. time: 5 min | Cooking time: 0 min | Servings: 2

INGREDIENTS:

- 4 slices white sandwich bread
- 2 lettuce leaves
- 2 tablespoons low-fat mayonnaise
- ½ can (from a 4 ounces can) low-sodium tuna packed in water, drained, rinsed

NUTRITIONAL VALUES PER SERVING: 1 SANDWICH	
Calories	318
Fat	13 g
Carbohydrates	37 g
Protein	10 g
Sodium	569 mg
Potassium	142 mg
Phosphorus	120 mg

DIRECTIONS:

1. Combine tuna and mayonnaise in a bowl. Spread the mixture onto 2 of the bread slices.
2. Place a lettuce leaf on each bread slice. Cover with the remaining 2 slices.
3. Cut into the desired shape and serve.

89. CRISPY CUCUMBER SALAD

Prep. time: 10 min | Cooking time: 0 min | Servings: 2

INGREDIENTS:

- 2 cups sliced cucumber (peeled or unpeeled)
- Freshly ground black pepper to taste
- 1 tablespoon Italian dressing or Caesar dressing

NUTRITIONAL VALUES PER SERVING: ½ CUP	
Calories	27
Fat	2 g
Carbohydrates	3 g
Protein	0 g
Sodium	74 mg
Potassium	14 mg
Phosphorus	14 mg

DIRECTIONS:

1. Place cucumber in a bowl. Add dressing and stir. Sprinkle pepper on top.
2. Cover the bowl and chill until use.

90. EGGPLANT KASHA

Prep. time: 15 min | Cooking time: 20 min | Servings: 2

INGREDIENTS:

- ½ cup roasted buckwheat groats (kasha)
- 1 ½ tablespoons olive oil, divided
- 1 clove garlic, minced
- 2 cups cubed eggplant
- 1 tablespoon pine nuts
- ¼ teaspoon capers
- ½ tablespoon pomegranate molasses
- ⅛ cup chopped parsley
- A tiny pinch black pepper
- ¾ cup water
- ½ medium yellow onion, chopped
- 1 stalk celery, chopped
- ½ small plum tomato, chopped
- ½ tablespoon pitted sliced black olives
- 1 tablespoon balsamic vinegar
- ⅛ cup chopped chives
- A pinch sea salt

NUTRITIONAL VALUES
PER SERVING: 1 CUP

Calories	322
Fat	14 g
Carbohydrates	46 g
Protein	7 g
Sodium	133 mg
Potassium	558 mg
Phosphorus	778 mg

DIRECTIONS:

1. Cook buckwheat groats and water in a saucepan. When water begins to boil, lower the heat and cook covered until dry and tender. Turn off the heat.
2. Pour 1 tablespoon of oil into a skillet and heat over medium-high heat. When oil is hot, add onion and cook until light brown.
3. Stir in garlic, eggplant, and celery and mix well. Cook until the eggplant is soft and a bit light brown in color.
4. Stir in olives, pine nuts, tomatoes, and capers and cook for a couple of minutes.
5. Turn off the heat and let it cool for 10 minutes.
6. Place the eggplant mixture in a blender. Add remaining oil and blend until slightly chunky.
7. Pour into a bowl. Add buckwheat groats and mix well.

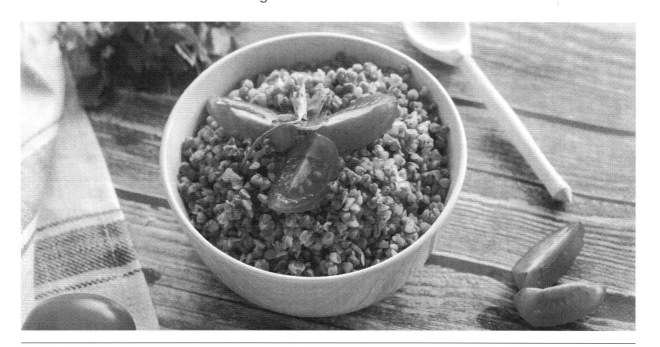

91. CHICKEN N' ORANGE SALAD SANDWICH

Prep. time: 10 min | Cooking time: 0 min | Servings: 3

INGREDIENTS:

- ½ cup cooked, cubed chicken
- ¼ cup diced green bell pepper
- ½ cup peeled, deseeded Mandarin orange segments
- ⅛ cup thinly sliced onion
- ¼ cup diced celery
- 3 tablespoons mayonnaise— Refer to Vegetarian Reuben sandwich for the mayonnaise recipe

NUTRITIONAL VALUES PER SERVING: ⅓ RECIPE (without serving option)	
Calories	162
Fat	10 g
Carbohydrates	6 g
Protein	10 g
Sodium	93 mg
Potassium	241 mg
Phosphorus	106 mg

DIRECTIONS:

1. Combine celery, chicken, onion, and green bell pepper in a bowl.
2. Fold in the oranges and mayonnaise.
3. Serve as a filling between 2 bread slices as a sandwich or over lettuce leaves or over wraps.

92. SUMMER VEGETABLE PANINI

Prep. time: 10 min | Cooking time: 20 min | Servings: 2

INGREDIENTS:

- ½ medium zucchini, halved lengthwise, cut into ½ inch thick slices crosswise
- 1 small onion, cut into ½ inch thick round slices
- ½ medium red bell pepper, cut into 2 halves
- 1 teaspoon balsamic vinegar
- A pinch salt
- A pinch pepper
- ¼ cup low-sodium homemade pesto
- ½ medium yellow squash, halved lengthwise, cut into ½ inch thick crosswise
- 2 ciabatta rolls, split

NUTRITIONAL VALUES PER SERVING: 1 SANDWICH	
Calories	480
Fat	29.1 g
Carbohydrates	47.2 g
Protein	11.9 g
Sodium	546.8 mg
Potassium	439.2 mg
Phosphorus	83.6 mg

DIRECTIONS:

1. Set up your grill and preheat it to medium heat.
2. Press the bell pepper to make it flat. Place the vegetables in a bowl. Drizzle a tablespoon of oil and vinegar over the vegetables. Sprinkle salt, pepper, and oregano over the vegetables and toss well.
3. Place the vegetables on the gill. Grill for 3-4 minutes. Turn the vegetables over and cook the other side for 3-4 minutes.
4. Spread a tablespoon of pesto on the cut side of each ciabatta. Divide the grilled vegetable and place on the bottom half of the ciabatta.
5. Cover the sandwich with the top half of the ciabatta rolls.
6. Grill the sandwich either on the grill or on a preheated panini press. In case you are grilling on the grill, place something heavy over the sandwiches to press them.
7. Grill to the desired doneness.

93. PEAS AND RAISINS PULAV

Prep. time: 12-15 min | Cooking time: 30-40 min | Servings: 6

INGREDIENTS:

- 1 ½ cups long grain white rice like basmati or jasmine, rinsed well, drained
- 4 tablespoons oil
- 2 teaspoons green chili pepper, deseeded, minced
- 1 teaspoon cumin seeds
- 6 tablespoons raisins
- 1 teaspoon turmeric powder
- ¼ cup chopped fresh basil or 2 teaspoons dried basil
- ½ teaspoon dried thyme
- 1 teaspoon dried oregano
- ½ teaspoon chili powder or to taste
- 1 cup frozen peas
- ⅓ cup cashews or almonds
- 2 teaspoons peeled, minced fresh ginger
- 2 ½ cups water
- 1 teaspoon salt or to taste
- ¼ teaspoon garam masala (Indian spice blend) or any other spice blend of your choice

NUTRITIONAL VALUES PER SERVING: ⅙ RECIPE (without yogurt)	
Calories	143
Fat	15.9 g
Carbohydrates	16.6 g
Protein	4.33 g
Sodium	419.79 mg
Potassium	252.88 mg
Phosphorus	137 mg

DIRECTIONS:

1. Place the rack in the center of the oven. Set the temperature of the oven to 375°F and preheat the oven.
2. Pour oil into a pot and place the pot over medium heat. Once the oil gets hot, drop the cashews or almonds into the pot and stir-fry until they turn light golden brown.
3. Take them out using a slotted spoon and place it on a plate layered with paper towels.
4. While the nuts are cooling, add cumin into the pot. In a few seconds, the cumin seeds will crackle.
5. Add ginger, turmeric, and green chili and stir constantly for about half a minute. Add rice and mix well. Stir often for a couple of minutes until the rice is well heated.
6. Add raisins, basil, thyme, salt, chili powder, oregano, and garam masala and mix well for 1-2 minutes.
7. Pour water and stir. Once it starts boiling, turn off the heat and transfer the contents of the pot into an ovenproof container. Keep the container covered tightly and place it in the oven.
8. Set the timer for 25 minutes. After about 20 minutes of cooking, uncover and scatter peas on top. Cover it once again and continue baking for the remaining 5 minutes.
9. Take out the baking dish from the oven and let it rest for 5-10 minutes on your countertop.
10. Uncover the dish and mix the peas into the rice using a fork.
11. Add the nuts and stir. Serve as it is or with yogurt.

94. CARAMELIZED ONION OPEN STEAK SANDWICH

Prep. time: 10 min | Cooking time: 10 min | Servings: 2

INGREDIENTS:

- 1 tablespoon olive oil
- ½ brown onion, sliced
- 1 teaspoon brown sugar
- 2 minute beef steaks (4 ounces each)
- 1 tablespoon horseradish cream
- A handful baby rocket leaves
- 0.4 ounce unsalted butter
- ½ teaspoon minced thyme leaves
- ½ tablespoon balsamic vinegar
- 1 small French baguette, halved lengthwise
- 4 slices cheddar cheese

NUTRITIONAL VALUES PER SERVING: 1 SANDWICH

Calories	388
Fat	30.81 g
Carbohydrates	11.66 g
Protein	15.81 g
Sodium	429.45 mg
Potassium	172.8 mg
Phosphorus	115 mg

DIRECTIONS:

1. Combine ½ tablespoon oil and butter in a nonstick pan. Place the pan over low heat and wait for the butter to melt.
2. When butter melts, add thyme and onion and cook until onions are soft.
3. Stir in vinegar and sugar and cook for some more time until the onions turn golden brown. Take the pan off heat.
4. While the onions are cooking, place another nonstick pan over medium heat. Add ½ tablespoon oil and let it heat.
5. Once oil is hot, place steaks in the pan and let it cook for 1-2 minutes on each side or cook the way you prefer it. Turn off the heat.
6. Smear ½ tablespoon horseradish cream on the cut part on each half of the baguette.
7. Place a steak on each baguette. Place 2 cheese slices on each.
8. Set the oven to broil mode and preheat the oven.
9. Place the sandwiches in the oven and broil for a few minutes until the cheese melts and is brown at a few spots.

95. CRUNCHY CHICKEN SALAD WRAPS

Prep. time: 10 min | Cooking time: 0 min | Servings: 2

INGREDIENTS:

- 4 ounces cooked chicken, shredded
- ¼ cup halved seedless grapes
- 2 tablespoons low sodium mayonnaise (refer to previous recipe to make low-sodium
- mayonnaise)
- 2 large lettuce leaves
- 1 small scallion, chopped
- ½ celery stalk, chopped
- A pinch freshly ground black pepper

NUTRITIONAL VALUES PER SERVING: 1 SANDWICH

Calories	147
Fat	5 g
Carbohydrates	8 g
Protein	15 g
Sodium	59 mg
Potassium	210 mg
Phosphorus	124 mg

DIRECTIONS:

1. Place chicken, celery, grapes, and scallions in a bowl and toss well. Add mayonnaise and fold gently.
2. Add pepper and mix gently.
3. Divide the chicken salad equally among the lettuce leaves and serve.

96. VEGETARIAN REUBEN SANDWICH

Prep. time: 15 min | Cooking time: 15 min | Servings: 1

INGREDIENTS:

- ½ large beet
- ¼ teaspoon freshly ground pepper
- 1 teaspoon olive oil
- ⅛ teaspoon finely crushed coriander seeds
- ½ tablespoon tomato paste
- ½ tablespoon fresh lemon juice
- 1 hot dog bun
- 1 slice low-sodium Swiss cheese

- ½ cornichon (small pickled cucumber), chopped
- ¾ teaspoon unsalted butter, softened
- 1 ¼ tablespoons sauerkraut, drained, warmed

MAYONNAISE:
- 1 small egg
- ½ cup sunflower oil or vegetable oil of your choice
- 1 teaspoon fresh lemon juice
- A pinch of sea salt

NUTRITIONAL VALUES PER SERVING: 1 CUP	
Calories	433
Fat	30 g
Carbohydrates	31 g
Protein	12 g
Sodium	394 mg
Potassium	172 mg
Phosphorus	172 mg

DIRECTIONS:

1. To make mayonnaise: Blend together eggs, salt, and lemon juice in a blender. With the blender machine running on medium speed, pour oil in a thin stream.
2. Increase the speed to high speed once the mayonnaise starts getting thick.
3. Pour into a jar and chill until use. It can last for 8-10 days.
4. To make sandwich filling: Cook beet in a pot of water until tender. Drain the water and set aside to cool. Once cooled, peel off the skin from the beet. Cut into ¼ inch thick slices.
5. Place beets on a plate. Pour a teaspoon of oil over the beets. Season with pepper and coriander seeds.
6. To make Russian dressing: Combine mayonnaise, cornichon, tomato paste, and lemon juice in a bowl.
7. Set the oven to broil mode and preheat the oven. Place the hot dog bun halves on a baking sheet with the cut side on top. Brush the bun halves with melted butter and place the baking sheet in the oven. Broil for a couple of minutes until it is toasted lightly.
8. Spread the Russian dressing over the bottom half of the bun. Remove the top half of the bun and set it aside.
9. Place beet slices and spread sauerkraut. Place the cheese slice on top and place the baking sheet back in the oven and broil for another 2 minutes or until the cheese melts.
10. Cover the sandwich by placing the top half of the sandwich. Cut into 2 halves and serve.

97. TORTILLA ROLL UPS

Prep. time: 10 min | Cooking time: 0 min | Servings: 2

INGREDIENTS:

- ¼ cup raw spinach leaves
- 1 tablespoon pimento
- ¼ cup crushed pineapple
- 1 low-sodium flour tortilla (burrito size)
- 1 tablespoon chopped onion
- 1.5 ounces unprocessed cooked turkey breast
- ¼ cup whipped cream cheese
- ½ teaspoon Mrs. Dash original herb seasoning blend

NUTRITIONAL VALUES PER SERVING	
Calories	223
Fat	11 g
Carbohydrates	21 g
Protein	10 g
Sodium	298 mg
Potassium	199 mg
Phosphorus	126 mg

DIRECTIONS:

1. Take cream cheese and spread it over the tortilla.
2. Dust the herb seasoning blend over the tortilla.
3. Combine onion, turkey, pimento, pineapple, and spinach in a bowl and place it on the bottom third part of the tortilla. Roll it up and place it with its seam side facing down.
4. Cut into 3-4 pieces and serve.

98. CHIPOTLE SHRIMP TACOS

Prep. time: 20 min | Cooking time: 4-5 min | Servings: 2

INGREDIENTS:

PINEAPPLE SALSA:
- ½ cup chopped pineapple
- ½ tablespoon chopped red onion
- ½ tablespoon lime juice
- 1 tablespoon chopped green onion
- 1 tablespoon chopped cilantro

SHRIMP TACOS:
- 2 tablespoons olive oil
- ¾ tablespoon southwest chipotle Mrs. Dash seasoning
- 2 corn tortillas (taco size)
- 1 clove garlic, minced
- 1 cup shredded cabbage
- ¾ pound shrimp, peeled, deveined, without tail, cooked (around 16 medium size shrimp)

NUTRITIONAL VALUES PER SERVING: 1 OVER-FILLED TACO	
Calories	250
Fat	14.4 g
Carbohydrates	22 g
Protein	29.9 g
Sodium	65 mg
Potassium	312 mg
Phosphorus	190 mg

DIRECTIONS:

1. Combine oil, garlic, shrimp, and Mrs. Dash seasoning in a bowl. Cover the bowl and keep it aside for about 10 minutes.
2. To make salsa: Combine all the salsa ingredients in a bowl. Keep the salsa aside for a while for the flavors to infuse.
3. Place a nonstick skillet over medium heat. When the pan is hot, add shrimp into the pan and cook for around 2 minutes.
4. Turn the shrimp over and cook for another 2 minutes.
5. To build the tacos: Divide the shrimp equally and place over the tortillas.
6. Place ½ cup cabbage over the shrimp on each tortilla.
7. Divide the salsa among the tortillas and serve.

99. ROASTED ASPARAGUS AND WILD MUSHROOM STEW

Prep. time: 40 min | Cooking time: 30-35 min | Servings: 2/3 cups

INGREDIENTS:

- ½ cup very hot water
- 1 celery stalk, chopped
- ½ small onion, chopped
- 2 sprigs fresh thyme
- Ground black pepper to taste
- ½ bay leaf
- A pinch onion powder
- 1 ounce pine nuts
- ½ fennel bulb, diced
- A pinch cayenne pepper
- ¾ tablespoon dry marsala wine
- ½ teaspoon dried sage
- ½ ounce dried wild mushroom medley
- 1 teaspoon olive oil + some cooking spray
- A pinch garlic powder
- 1 cup low-sodium vegetable stock
- ½ pound asparagus, trim the tough ends
- ½ tablespoon chopped parsley

NUTRITIONAL VALUES PER SERVING: 1 CUP	
Calories	103
Fat	5.8 g
Carbohydrates	11.7 g
Protein	3.4 g
Sodium	78.8 mg
Potassium	436.8 mg
Phosphorus	69.8 mg

DIRECTIONS:

1. Place mushrooms into the cup with hot water. Let it rehydrate for about 30-40 minutes.
2. Set the temperature of your oven to 400°F and preheat the oven.
3. Lay the asparagus spears on a baking sheet without overlapping.
4. Spray a bit of boil over the spears. Place the baking sheet in the oven and let the timer be set for 10 minutes. Once the asparagus cools down, chop them into 1 inch pieces.
5. Pour oil into a nonstick pan and place the pan over medium-high heat.
6. Add the vegetables and cook until the onion turns pink.
7. Stir in sage, thyme, cayenne pepper, parsley, bay leaf, onion powder, wine, and garlic powder.
8. Stir constantly for 1 minute.
9. Pour the stock and soaked mushroom water and stir. Add the mushrooms (chop into pieces before adding) as well.
10. Cook on low heat for about 15 minutes. Serve asparagus and stew in bowls garnished with pine nuts.

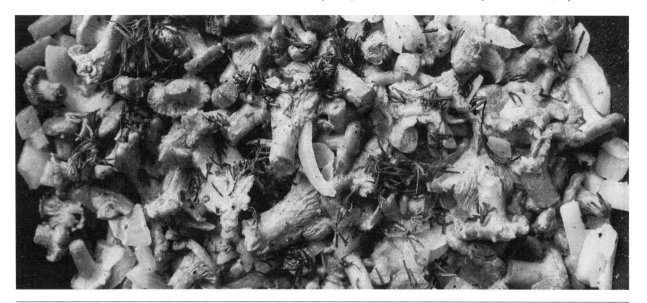

100. ZUCCHINI BREAD

Prep. time: 15 min | Cooking time: 40 min | Servings: 5

INGREDIENTS:

- 1 egg
- ⅓ cup applesauce
- ⅓ teaspoon vanilla extract
- ⅓ teaspoon baking soda
- A pinch baking powder
- ⅓ teaspoon ground cinnamon
- ⅓ cup chopped nuts
- ½ cup sugar
- ⅔ cup unpeeled, shredded zucchini
- ⅔ cup flour
- ⅛ teaspoon ground ginger

NUTRITIONAL VALUES PER SERVING: 1 SLICE	
Calories	200
Fat	6.4 g
Carbohydrates	33.2 g
Protein	4.4 g
Sodium	100 mg
Potassium	128 mg
Phosphorus	78 mg

DIRECTIONS:

1. Crack egg into a bowl and beat well.
2. Add vanilla, sugar, zucchini, and applesauce and mix well.
3. Sift together flour, baking powder, cinnamon, ginger, and baking soda in a bowl.
4. Add the flour mixture into the bowl of zucchini and stir until just incorporated.
5. Grease a small loaf pan with a little oil. Spoon the batter into the loaf pan.
6. Preheat the oven to 375°F.
7. Place the loaf pan in the oven and bake for about 40-50 minutes or until cooked through and golden brown on top. Check if the bread is cooked by inserting a toothpick in the center of the bread. Remove it and check if there are any particles stuck on it. If you see any particles stuck on it, bake it for a few more minutes, otherwise turn off your oven and remove the loaf pan.
8. Cut into 5 equal slices and serve.

101. MEXICAN STYLE STUFFED PEPPERS

Prep. time: 30 min | Cooking time: 60 min | Servings: 4

INGREDIENTS:

- 2 red bell peppers, cut into 2 halves lengthwise
- ¾ pound 93% lean ground turkey
- 2 tablespoons finely chopped cilantro
- 3 cup cooked brown rice
- ⅓ cup +2 tablespoons fresh salsa
- 1 small egg
- ¼ teaspoon ground black pepper
- ⅓ cup finely chopped onion
- ½ tablespoon chili powder

NUTRITIONAL VALUES PER SERVING: ½ STUFFED PEPPER	
Calories	226.8
Fat	10 g
Carbohydrates	12 g
Protein	23 g
Sodium	122 mg
Potassium	483 mg
Phosphorus	258 mg

DIRECTIONS:

1. Preheat the oven to 350°F.
2. Deseed and remove membranes from the bell peppers.
3. Combine rice, ⅓ cup salsa, turkey, onion, chili powder, pepper, cilantro, and egg in a bowl.
4. Divide the filling among the bell peppers and place in a baking dish. Pour ⅛ cup water around the bell peppers in the baking dish. Cover the baking dish with foil.
5. Place the baking sheet in the oven and bake for 45 minutes. Remove the foil and place ½ tablespoon salsa on top of each bell pepper. Continue baking for another 15 minutes.

102. ROASTED ONION GARLIC PIZZA

Prep. time: 60 min | Cooking time: 45 min | Servings: 3 cups

INGREDIENTS:

- ¼ teaspoon dried rosemary
- 3 teaspoons sugar
- 1 ½ cups all-purpose flour
- 1 ounce warm water
- 1 head garlic, peel the cloves
- 1 tablespoon canola oil
- ¾ cup unenriched rice milk
- ½ packet Baker's active dry yeast
- 2 ½ medium red onions, sliced

NUTRITIONAL VALUES PER SERVING: 1 CUP	
Calories	180
Fat	3 g
Carbohydrates	34 g
Protein	4.4 g
Sodium	13 mg
Potassium	116 mg
Phosphorus	73 mg

DIRECTIONS:

1. Combine yeast and warm water in a mixing bowl and keep it aside for 5 minutes.
2. Add sugar, rice milk, oil, and flour and mix well. Mix until dough is formed. You can do it with your hand or with the stand mixer with the dough hook attachment.
3. Knead the dough for 8-10 minutes.
4. Grease a bowl with a generous amount of oil. Place dough in the bowl. Turn the dough around in the bowl to grease the dough as well.
5. Keep the bowl covered with cling wrap and keep it in a warm place for about 30-40 minutes or until it doubles in size.
6. Meanwhile, prepare the pizza toppings: Preheat the oven to 350°F.
7. Place onion on a greased baking sheet. Spray the onion with cooking spray. Wrap garlic in foil and place on the baking sheet next to the onions. Place the baking sheet in the oven and roast for 30-40 minutes. Stir the onions every 10-15 minutes and bake until brown.
8. By now, the dough would have doubled in size. Cut into 3 equal portions and shape into balls.
9. Roll or pat the dough balls into the shape of a pizza, to the thickness you desire. Place the rolled dough on a baking sheet.
10. Scatter roasted garlic, onion, and rosemary over the pizza dough.
11. Bake for 12-15 minutes. Cut into wedges and serve.

103. VERY BERRY TOFU SMOOTHIE

Prep. time: 10 min | Cooking time: 0 min | Servings: 3-4

INGREDIENTS:

- ½ pound fresh strawberries, cleaned, hulled
- 4.5 ounces tofu, silken, extra-firm
- A pinch red pepper flakes
- ½ tablespoon honey
- ¼ cup ice
- 1 cup blueberries
- ¼ teaspoon ground ginger
- ⅛ teaspoon rum extract
- ½ teaspoon lemon juice

NUTRITIONAL VALUES PER SERVING: 1 CUP	
Calories	136
Fat	2.4 g
Carbohydrates	25.7 g
Protein	5.8 g
Sodium	25.7 mg
Potassium	365.8 mg
Phosphorus	94.8 mg

DIRECTIONS:

1. Blend together berries, tofu, spices, rum extract, and lemon juice in a blender and blend until smooth.
2. Add ice and blend until very chilled. Pour into cups and serve.

104. BAKED SEA BASS

Prep. time: 15 min | Cooking time: 20 min | Servings: 2

INGREDIENTS:

NUTRITIONAL VALUES PER SERVING: 1 CUP	
Calories	380
Calcium	16 g
Protein	24 g
Sodium	74 mg
Potassium	279 mg
Phosphorus	211 mg

- 2 Sea Bass fillets
- 2 small potatoes
- 1 onion
- 1 large carrot
- 1 red pepper
- 2 tablespoon fresh basil
- 1 tablespoon olive oil

DIRECTIONS:

1. Cook the potatoes in a pan of boiling water until they are soft. Once cooked remove from water and let them cool, then dice them. Cut the peppers into strips, peel and slice the carrot and onion.
2. In a non-stick frying pan heat the olive oil over medium-high heat and add the fillets.
3. Sear each side for about 4 minutes. Once cooked remove and place on a plate. Cover to keep the fish warm. Add the onion, carrot and red pepper to the frying pan and sauté for 5 minutes, until softened. Add the mix to the fish plate. Serve the sea bass with the potatoes, finishing with a sprinkle of basil.

105. BUCKWHEAT WITH MUSHROOMS

Prep. time: 15 min | Cooking time: 30 min | Servings: 3

INGREDIENTS:

NUTRITIONAL VALUES PER SERVING: 1 SANDWICH	
Calories	168
Fat	5 g
Carbohydrates	27 g
Protein	7 g
Sodium	46 mg
Potassium	470 mg
Phosphorus	138 mg

- ½ cup uncooked buckwheat
- 8 ounces mushrooms
- ½ cup green onion, diced
- 1 cup water
- ½ medium onion, chopped
- 1 ½ tablespoons unsalted butter
- Ground pepper to taste

DIRECTIONS:

Combine water and buckwheat in a saucepan. Place the saucepan over medium heat. When water starts boiling, lower the heat and cook until dry. Turn off the heat. Melt butter in a pan. Add onion to the melted butter and sauté until golden brown. Add cooked buckwheat and mix well. Turn off the heat. Let it sit covered for 10 minutes. Stir in green onion. Divide equally into 3 plates and serve.

106. ROCKET AND CHICKPEA SALAD

Prep. time: 5 min | Cooking time: 0 min | Servings: 2

INGREDIENTS:

NUTRITIONAL VALUES PER SERVING	
Calories	194
Calcium	20 g
Protein	15 g
Sodium	18 mg
Potassium	192 mg
Phosphorus	78 mg

- 4 cups of rocket leaves
- ½ cup canned chickpeas
- 3 tablespoons olive oil
- 2 tablespoons lemon juice
- ½ teaspoon mustard

DIRECTIONS:

Wash the rocket leaves. In a small bowl whisk the olive oil, lemon juice and mustard. Place rocket leaves in a mixing bowl and drizzle the dressing over it. Add the chickpeas, mix and serve.

107. SESAME AND GINGER SOBA NOODLES

Prep. time: 15 min | Cooking time: 15-20 min | Servings: 3 cups

INGREDIENTS:

- 1 cup thinly sliced cabbage
- ¼ cup thinly sliced green onions
- 2 cloves garlic, minced
- ⅛ cup chopped cilantro
- ½ cup broccoli florets, steamed
- ¼ cup diced red bell pepper
- ⅛ cup minced shallots
- 1 tablespoon minced ginger
- ½ teaspoon sesame oil
- ½ tablespoon low-sodium soy sauce
- ¼ teaspoon sesame seeds
- A pinch red pepper flakes or to taste
- ½ tablespoon mirin
- 1 ¼ tablespoons canola oil
- ½ teaspoon brown sugar
- A pinch black pepper
- ½ package (from an 8 ounces package) soba noodles

NUTRITIONAL VALUES PER SERVING	
Calories	230
Fat	5 g
Carbohydrates	37 g
Protein	9 g
Sodium	188 mg
Potassium	284 mg
Phosphorus	65 mg

DIRECTIONS:

1. Make the sauce mixture by combining ginger, sesame oil, soy sauce, 1 tablespoon shallot, green onion, black pepper, ¾ tablespoon oil, brown sugar, half the garlic, sesame seeds, and red pepper flakes in a bowl. Whisk until well combined.
2. Cook the noodles in a pot of water over high heat until just al dente.
3. Drain and immerse in a bowl of cold running water. Drain well. Repeat this a few times until the noodles stop sticking to each other.
4. Pour remaining oil into a skillet and place the skillet over medium heat.
5. Stir the remaining onion and garlic into the oil in the skillet and cook for about a minute until you get a nice aroma.
6. Stir in cabbage, broccoli, and bell pepper and cook for a couple of minutes.
7. Add soba noodles and the sauce mixture and stir gently. Heat thoroughly.
8. Serve in bowls garnished with cilantro.

108. PEANUT BUTTER SANDWICH

Prep. time: 10 min | Cooking time: 0 min | Servings: 2 cups

NUTRITIONAL VALUES PER SERVING	
Calories	456
Fat	21 g
Carbohydrates	50 g
Protein	17 g
Sodium	510 mg
Potassium	489 mg
Phosphorus	322 mg

INGREDIENTS:

- 4 slices raisin bread
- 2 teaspoons honey
- 2 stalks celery, chopped
- 1 cup raspberries
- 3 tablespoons natural peanut butter
- 2 ounces string cheese, chopped

DIRECTIONS:

1. Spread 1 ½ tablespoons of peanut butter on each of 2 bread slices.
2. Spread a teaspoon of honey over each of them. Cover the sandwich with the remaining bread slices. Cut into the desired shape and serve with celery, raspberries, and cheese.

109. STUFFED ZUCCHINI BOATS

Prep. time: 15 min | Cooking time: 45 min | Servings: 1

INGREDIENTS:

- 1 medium zucchini, trimmed, halved lengthwise, scoop out some of the seeds using a spoon—these are the zucchini boats
- ½ teaspoon original Mrs. Dash seasoning blend
- ½ teaspoon dill weed
- ⅛ teaspoon ground sage
- 2 slices white bread, toasted
- ½ teaspoon onion powder
- ½ teaspoon salt-free lemon pepper

NUTRITIONAL VALUES PER SERVING: 1 ZUCCHINI BOAT	
Calories	82
Fat	1 g
Carbohydrates	15 g
Protein	3 g
Sodium	180 mg
Potassium	276 mg
Phosphorus	63 mg

DIRECTIONS:

1. Boil a pot of water over high heat. Add zucchini and drain off after 3-4 minutes, retaining about ½ cup of the cooked water. Do not overcook the zucchini; it should have a bit of crunch in it.
2. Set the temperature of your oven to 375°F and preheat the oven.
3. Tear the toasted bread slices and place in a blender. Process until breadcrumbs are formed.
4. Combine breadcrumbs, herbs, and spices in a bowl. Add 4-5 tablespoons of the cooked zucchini water and stir using a fork.
5. Fill this mixture into the zucchini boats. Place the baking sheet in the oven and set the timer for 20 minutes.

110. RANCH CHICKEN PASTA

Prep. time: 15 min | Cooking time: 30 min | Servings: 2-3

INGREDIENTS:

- 8 ounces penne pasta
- ½ tablespoon all-purpose white flour
- 1 teaspoon dried parsley flakes
- ¼ teaspoon garlic powder
- ¼ teaspoon dill weed
- A pinch pepper
- 1 cup cooked, cubed chicken breast
- ⅛ cup shredded parmesan cheese
- ½ cup reduced-fat sour cream
- ¼ cup shredded reduced-fat Mexican cheese blend
- ½ tablespoon butter
- ½ cup unenriched rice milk
- ½ teaspoon salt-free lemon pepper seasoning
- ¼ teaspoon dried minced onion
- ⅛ teaspoon onion powder

NUTRITIONAL VALUES PER SERVING: 1½ CUPS	
Calories	237
Fat	9 g
Carbohydrates	23 g
Protein	16 g
Sodium	150 mg
Potassium	184 mg
Phosphorus	204 mg

DIRECTIONS:

1. Drop pasta into a pot of boiling water and cook until al dente. Drain in a colander and keep it aside.
2. Melt butter in a heavy bottomed pan. Add flour and keep stirring until roux is formed.
3. Stir in rice milk and seasonings. Whisk constantly until smooth and thick.
4. Lower the heat and add sour cream. Stir until well combined.
5. Stir the pasta and chicken into the sauce. Cook for a couple of minutes and serve.

111. BBQ CHICKEN PITA PIZZA

Prep. time: 10 min | Cooking time: 13 min | Servings: 1

INGREDIENTS:

NUTRITIONAL VALUES PER SERVING	
Calories	320
Fat	9 g
Carbohydrates	37 g
Protein	23 g
Sodium	523 mg
Potassium	255 mg
Phosphorus	221 mg

- 1 pita bread (6 ½ inches)
- ⅛ cup diced purple onion
- 2 ounces cooked chicken
- 1 ½ tablespoons low-sodium
- BBQ sauce
- 1 tablespoon crumbled feta cheese
- A pinch garlic powder

DIRECTIONS:

1. Preheat the oven to 375°F.
2. Grease a baking sheet with some cooking spray. Spread BBQ sauce over the pita and place it on the baking sheet.
3. Scatter onion and chicken over the pita. Sprinkle garlic powder over the onion and chicken.
4. Sprinkle feta cheese on top and place the baking sheet in the oven and bake for 12-13 minutes.
5. Serve hot.

112. SHRIMP QUESADILLA

Prep. time: 15 min | Cooking time: 12-15 min | Servings: 1 cup

INGREDIENTS:

NUTRITIONAL VALUES PER SERVING	
Calories	318
Fat	15 g
Carbohydrates	26 g
Protein	20 g
Sodium	398 mg
Potassium	276 mg
Phosphorus	243 mg

- 2.5 ounces raw shrimp, shelled, deveined, cut into bite size pieces
- ½ tablespoon fresh lemon juice
- A pinch cayenne pepper
- 1 tablespoon sour cream
- 1 tablespoon shredded jalapeño cheddar cheese
- 1 tablespoon chopped cilantro
- ⅛ teaspoon ground cumin
- 1 flour tortilla (burrito size)
- 2 teaspoons salsa
- Lemon wedge to serve

DIRECTIONS:

1. Add cilantro, cumin, lemon juice, and cayenne pepper into a Ziploc bag. Shake the bag until well combined. Add shrimp into the bag. Seal the bag and turn it around a few times until shrimp is well coated. Let it sit for 5 minutes.
2. Place a skillet over medium heat. Add shrimp along with the marinade and sauté until shrimp is orange in color. Turn off the heat.
3. Remove shrimp with a slotted spoon and keep it on a plate. Do not discard the marinade.
4. Add sour cream into the skillet and mix well.
5. Spread salsa all over the tortilla. Place shrimp on one half of the tortilla. Scatter cheese over the shrimp.
6. Spread a little of the sour cream mixture over the shrimp. Fold the other half of the tortilla over the filling. Press slightly.
7. Place a nonstick pan over medium heat. Place the quesadilla in the pan. Cook until the underside is golden brown. Flip sides and cook the other side until golden brown.
8. Cut into pieces. Sprinkle cilantro on top and serve with a lemon wedge.

113. MEATLOAF

Prep. time: 5 min | Cooking time: 3 min | Servings: 2

INGREDIENTS:

NUTRITIONAL VALUES PER SERVING: 1 MUG	
Calories	252
Fat	10 g
Carbohydrates	13 g
Protein	25 g
Sodium	170 mg
Potassium	397 mg
Phosphorus	246 mg

- 4 tablespoons 1% low-fat milk
- 2 teaspoons onion powder
- 4 tablespoons quick cooking oats
- ½ pound lean ground beef, crumbled
- 4 teaspoons low-sodium ketchup

DIRECTIONS:

1. Grease 2 microwave safe mugs (12 ounces each) with some cooking spray.
2. Place oats, ketchup, onion powder, and milk in a bowl. Mix well.
3. Add beef and stir until well combined. Divide the mixture into the mugs
4. Place in a microwave and cook on High for 3 minutes or until the meat is not pink anymore.
5. Cool for a few minutes and serve.

114. VEGGIE STIR-FRY

Prep. time: 15 min | Cooking time: 5-8 min | Servings: 1

INGREDIENTS:

NUTRITIONAL VALUES PER SERVING	
Calories	231
Fat	9 g
Carbohydrates	13 g
Protein	14 g
Sodium	355 mg
Potassium	442 mg
Phosphorus	54 mg

- 6 ounces mixed greens, thinly shredded
- ¼ cup white wine vinegar or rice vinegar
- ½ tablespoon low-sodium soy sauce
- 4 ounces tofu, cut into cubes
- ¼ teaspoon sesame seeds
- ½ tablespoon olive oil
- ½ teaspoon sesame oil
- ⅛ teaspoon curry powder
- ½ cup thinly sliced onion

DIRECTIONS:

1. Pour olive oil into a pan and place the pan over high heat. When oil is hot, add onion and cook until soft. Add tofu, curry powder, sugar, and mixed greens and mix well.
2. Cover the pan and cook on low heat until the greens wilt. Take out the mixture with a slotted spoon and place on a plate.
3. Add soy sauce and vinegar into the pan and let it cook into a slightly thick sauce.
4. Turn off the heat. Spoon the sauce over the tofu and greens mixture. Drizzle sesame oil on top. Sprinkle sesame seeds on top and serve.

CHAPTER 9

Dinner Recipes

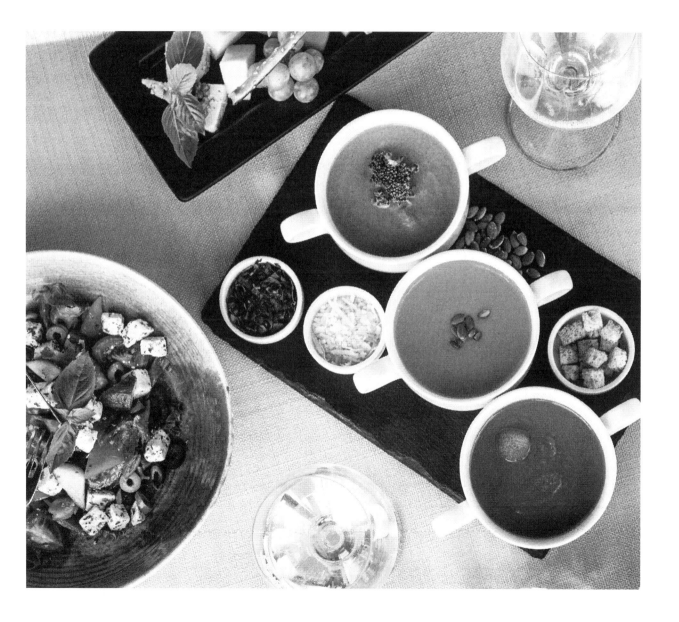

115. CHICKEN AND DUMPLINGS

Prep. time: 15 min | Cooking time: 20 min | Servings: 3

INGREDIENTS:

- 2 small bay leaves
- ⅛ teaspoon celery seeds
- ¼ teaspoon dried thyme
- Pepper to taste
- ½ tablespoon dried parsley
- ¼ teaspoon dried rosemary
- 1 drop sriracha sauce
- ½ stalk celery, thinly sliced
- ½ small yellow onion, minced
- 1 carrot, cut into ½ inch cubes
- ½ teaspoon baking powder
- ¾ cup cooked, diced chicken
- 1 tablespoon chopped fresh parsley + extra to garnish
- 2 ½ tablespoons cold, unsalted butter, divided
- 1 ½ cups low-sodium chicken broth
- 5.3 ounces green beans, trimmed, cut into 1 inch pieces
- ¼ cup unenriched rice milk or almond milk
- ½ cup + ⅛ cup all-purpose flour, divided
- Spices of your choice if desired

NUTRITIONAL VALUES PER SERVING: 1 CUP	
Calories	283
Fat	13 g
Carbohydrates	26.8 g
Protein	14.3 g
Sodium	186 mg
Potassium	478.6 mg
Phosphorus	282.7 mg

DIRECTIONS:

1. Add 1 ½ tablespoons of butter into a saucepan. Place the saucepan over medium-high heat.
2. Once butter melts, add celery, onion, and carrot and cook until onion turns pink.
3. Stir in ⅛ cup flour, bay leaves, celery seeds, and dried herb into the vegetable mixture. Stir constantly for about a minute. Add broth and keep stirring until slightly thick.
4. When it starts boiling, lower the heat and cook for 3-4 minutes.
5. Add green beans, chicken, and pepper and mix well.
6. Make the dumplings: Combine baking powder, ½ cup flour, and fresh parsley in a bowl. Add butter and cut it into the flour mixture using a pastry cutter of your hand.
7. Add almond milk and stir. Take a spoonful of batter and drop it into the saucepan over the chicken. Repeat this and try to cover the top of the chicken with the batter.
8. Cover the saucepan and cook until vegetables and dumplings are cooked.

116. HEARTY CHICKEN SOUP

Prep. time: 10-12 min | Cooking time: 25 min | Servings: 4 cup

INGREDIENTS:

- ¾ cup sliced celery
- ¾ cup chopped onion
- ½ cup cubed carrots
- 1 cup frozen green peas
- ½ tablespoon olive oil
- 1 teaspoon dried basil
- ½ teaspoon dried oregano
- ½ teaspoon dried thyme
- ¼ cup 1% low-fat milk
- ⅛ teaspoon pepper

- ½ cup fresh beans, trimmed, cut into ½ inch pieces
- ⅛ teaspoon ground nutmeg
- 1 cup low-sodium chicken broth
- 1 ½ tablespoons all-purpose flour
- ½ pound boneless, skinless chicken breasts

NUTRITIONAL VALUES PER SERVING: 1½ CUPS	
Calories	131
Fat	3 g
Carbohydrates	12 g
Protein	14 g
Sodium	343 mg
Potassium	467 mg
Phosphorus	171 mg

DIRECTIONS:

1. Pour oil into a soup pot and place the pot over medium heat. Add onion and celery and cook for 3-4 minutes.
2. Stir in chicken and cook for a couple of minutes. Add carrots, flour, beans, and seasonings and stir well.
3. Pour milk and broth and stir well. When it starts boiling, lower the heat and simmer until chicken is cooked.
4. Add peas and stir. Turn off the heat after about 5 minutes. Stir in pepper and serve.

117. HONEY GARLIC CHICKEN

Prep. time: 5 min | Cooking time: 45 min | Servings: 2

INGREDIENTS:

- 2 pounds roasting chicken, cut into pieces
- ½ teaspoon garlic powder
- ½ tablespoon olive oil
- ¼ cup honey
- ¼ teaspoon pepper

NUTRITIONAL VALUES PER SERVING	
Calories	279
Fat	10 g
Carbohydrates	36 g
Protein	13 g
Sodium	40 mg
Potassium	144 mg
Phosphorus	99 mg

DIRECTIONS:

1. Preheat the oven to 350°F. Prepare a baking dish by greasing it with some oil. Place chicken in the baking dish without overlapping.
2. Brush with honey all over the chicken. Sprinkle garlic powder and pepper.
3. Place the baking dish in the oven and set the timer for about 45 minutes or until brown and cooked through. Turn the chicken over half way through baking. Serve hot.

118. CHINESE CHICKEN SALAD

Prep. time: 10 min | Cooking time: 5 min | Servings: 4

INGREDIENTS:

- 1 package ramen noodles
- 1 tablespoon sesame seeds
- ¼ head cabbage, shredded
- 2 tablespoons sugar or splenda
- ¼ cup white vinegar or rice vinegar
- 1 ½ tablespoons olive oil, divided
- 1 cup cooked, diced chicken or turkey
- 2 green onions, sliced
- ½ tablespoon sesame oil

NUTRITIONAL VALUES PER SERVING: 1 CUP	
Calories	203
Fat	3.5 g
Carbohydrates	13 g
Protein	19 g
Sodium	48 mg
Potassium	259 mg
Phosphorus	41 mg

DIRECTIONS:

1. Take a rolling pin and beat the unopened package of noodles to break the noodles.
2. Now open the package. Do not use the seasoning packet that comes with the ramen noodles. Use seasoning of your choice that is renal diet friendly.
3. To make dressing: Whisk together 1 tablespoon olive oil, sugar, vinegar, and sesame oil in a bowl. Whisk until sugar dissolves.
4. Pour ½ tablespoon olive oil into a skillet and let it heat. Add the noodles and sesame seeds and cook until golden brown, stirring often.
5. Turn off the heat and let it cool.
6. Combine cabbage, chicken, and green onion in a bowl. Add noodles just before serving and toss well. Pour dressing on top. Toss well and serve.

119. CHICKEN FRUIT SALAD

Prep. time: 10 min | Cooking time: 0 min + chilling time | Servings: 3-4

NUTRITIONAL VALUES PER SERVING: 1⅓ CUPS	
Calories	380
Fat	21 g
Carbohydrates	31 g
Protein	17 g
Sodium	183 mg
Potassium	291 mg
Phosphorus	159 mg

INGREDIENTS:

- 4 ounces uncooked small shell pasta
- ¾ cup sliced celery
- ½ can (from a 15 ounces can) mandarin oranges
- 1 ½ cups cooked chicken
- ¾ cup halved seedless grapes
- 6 tablespoons mayonnaise— refer Vegetarian Reuben sandwich for the recipe

DIRECTIONS:

1. Cook pasta in a pot of water over medium-high heat until al dente. Drain the pasta and rinse well under cold running water. Place it in a colander for 5 minutes.
2. Add pasta, mayonnaise, chicken, celery, and oranges in a bowl. Stir well and cover the bowl.
3. Chill until use.

120. MEDITERRANEAN CHICKEN AND PASTA

Prep. time: 10 min | Cooking time: 30-40 min | Servings: 4 cup

INGREDIENTS:

- ½ teaspoon dried basil
- ⅛ teaspoon dried rosemary
- ¼ teaspoon dried oregano
- 1 cup dry pasta
- ¼ teaspoon freshly ground black pepper
- ¼ cup red or white wine
- 1 teaspoon cornstarch
- 1 tablespoon chopped fresh parsley to garnish
- 1 tomato, cut into ½ inch cubes
- 2 cloves garlic, minced
- ½ tablespoon olive oil
- 1 ¼ cups low-sodium chicken broth
- 1 ½ tablespoons shredded parmesan cheese
- 1 medium zucchini, halved lengthwise, cut into slices crosswise
- ½ medium red bell pepper, cut into ½ inch squares
- 1 medium chicken breast (about 7 ounces), skinless, boneless, chopped into bite size chunks

NUTRITIONAL VALUES PER SERVING	
Calories	245
Fat	4.4 g
Carbohydrates	26 g
Protein	4.4 g
Sodium	84 mg
Potassium	436 mg
Phosphorus	222 mg

DIRECTIONS:

1. Pour oil into a pot and place it over medium-high heat. When oil is hot, add chicken and cook until light brown all over.
2. Stir in tomato, zucchini, garlic, and bell pepper. Add herbs and pepper and mix well. Cook until the vegetables are crisp as well as tender. Turn off the heat.
3. Combine broth and wine in another pot and heat it over medium-high heat. When the mixture starts boiling, add pasta and cook until just tender. Turn off the heat.
4. Take out about ½ cup of liquid from the pot of pasta and pour into a bowl. Let it cool for 5 minutes. Add cornstarch and stir until smooth and free from lumps.
5. Transfer the pasta and the liquid in the pot into the pot of chicken. Mix well. Add cornstarch mixture.
6. Simmer for a few minutes until the sauce is slightly thick. Stir often.
7. Add parmesan cheese and stir. Turn off the heat.
8. Divide into 4 equal portions and serve garnished with parsley.

121. CHICKEN AND RICE CASSEROLE

Prep. time: 10 min | Cooking time: 50 min | Servings: 3

INGREDIENTS:

- ½ cup diced bell pepper
- 1 tablespoon olive oil
- 3 tablespoons all-purpose flour
- ½ tablespoon low-sodium Worcestershire sauce
- ½ cup 1% low-fat milk
- 1 cup cooked, cubed chicken
- ½ tablespoon Mrs. Dash herb seasoning blend
- ¼ cup chopped onion
- 1 tablespoon unsalted butter
- ⅛ teaspoon black pepper
- 1 ½ cups cooked white rice
- ½ cup sliced fresh mushrooms
- ½ cup low-sodium chicken broth

NUTRITIONAL VALUES PER SERVING: 1 CUP	
Calories	331
Fat	11 g
Carbohydrates	38 g
Protein	20 g
Sodium	125 mg
Potassium	386 mg
Phosphorus	216 mg

DIRECTIONS:

1. Preheat the oven to 350°F. Grease a baking dish with some cooking spray.
2. Pour oil into a skillet and place it over low heat. Add butter and allow it to melt.
3. Add flour and pepper and mix well. Stir until roux is formed. Take off the pan from heat.
4. Add Worcestershire sauce, milk, and broth and whisk well. Place the skillet back over heat and stir constantly until it starts boiling. Turn off the heat.
5. Add rice, vegetables, chicken, and seasoning and stir. Spoon the mixture into the baking dish.
6. Cover the dish with foil and place it in the oven. Set the timer for about 25 minutes.
7. Uncover and bake for 15-20 minutes.

122. CHICKEN AND PASTA

Prep. time: 5 min | Cooking time: 10 min | Servings: 1

INGREDIENTS:

- ½ tablespoon olive oil
- ½ cup sliced zucchini
- 2.5 ounces cooked chicken breast, cut into strips
- ¼ cup sliced red bell pepper
- 1 cup cooked pasta
- 1 ½ tablespoons low-sodium Italian dressing

NUTRITIONAL VALUES PER SERVING	
Calories	400
Fat	11 g
Carbohydrates	45 g
Protein	30 g
Sodium	328 mg
Potassium	455 mg
Phosphorus	270 mg

DIRECTIONS:

1. Pour oil into a skillet and heat it over medium heat. Add zucchini and bell pepper and cook for a few minutes until crisp as well as tender.
2. Warm the pasta in a microwave. Transfer into a bowl. Add dressing and stir.
3. Warm the chicken strips in the microwave. Place chicken over the pasta and serve.

123. BEEF BURGER

Prep. time: 5 min | Cooking time: 10-12 min | Servings: 2

INGREDIENTS:

- 1 ½ tablespoons un-enriched rice milk
- 1 small egg
- ½ pound 85% lean ground beef
- 2 ½ unsalted soda crackers, crushed
- ½ teaspoon salt free herb seasoning like Mrs. Dash

NUTRITIONAL VALUES PER SERVING: 1 BURGER (without serving options)	
Calories	242
Fat	14 g
Carbohydrates	7 g
Protein	22 g
Sodium	92 mg
Potassium	328 mg
Phosphorus	188 mg

DIRECTIONS:

1. Place crackers in a bowl. Add milk and stir. Set aside until the crackers are softened.
2. Stir in egg, herb seasoning, and beef. Mix with your hand until well combined, making sure not to over-mix.
3. Divide the mixture into 2 equal portions and shape into patties.
4. Cook the burgers either in a grill pan or on a preheated grill over medium heat on both the sides until the internal temperature of the burger when checked with a meat thermometer shows around 160°F.
5. Serve over buns or lettuce leaves with renal diet friendly toppings of your choice if desired.

124. SPAGHETTI WITH MEAT SAUCE

Prep. time: 5 min | Cooking time: 30-35 min | Servings: 4

INGREDIENTS:

- 4 ounces whole-wheat spaghetti, uncooked
- ½ cup diced onion
- ½ tablespoon Italian seasoning
- 7 ounces low sodium spaghetti sauce
- ¾ pound ground beef
- 3 tablespoons brown sugar
- ½ teaspoon garlic powder

NUTRITIONAL VALUES PER SERVING: 1 CUP	
Calories	317
Fat	9 g
Carbohydrates	36 g
Protein	23 g
Sodium	269 mg
Potassium	538 mg
Phosphorus	256 mg

DIRECTIONS:

1. Cook pasta in a pot of water over medium heat until al dente. Drain off the water and rinse under cold running water.
2. Add beef and onion into a pan and cook the meat mixture over medium heat, until brown. As you stir, break the meat. Discard any extra fat from the pan.
3. Stir in sugar, garlic powder, and Italian seasoning. Mix well and add the spaghetti sauce.
4. Cook for a few minutes until sugar dissolves completely. Add pasta and mix well.
5. Serve hot.

125. GROUND BEEF AND GREEN PEA CASSEROLE

Prep. time: 10 min | Cooking time: 30 min | Servings: 3

INGREDIENTS:

- 1 ½ cups new potatoes, peeled, cut into cubes
- ½ pound lean ground beef
- 1 ½ cups fresh shelled green peas
- 1 tablespoon cornstarch
- ½ medium onion, chopped
- 1 ¼ cups water + extra to cook potatoes
- 1 cup low-sodium beef broth

NUTRITIONAL VALUES PER SERVING: 1 CUP	
Calories	268
Fat	8 g
Carbohydrates	28 g
Protein	21 g
Sodium	154 mg
Potassium	632 mg
Phosphorus	270 mg

DIRECTIONS:

1. Place potatoes in a pot of water and place the pot over medium heat. When water starts boiling, drain the potatoes and place it back in the pot. Pour some water over the potatoes to cover them and place the pot over high heat.
2. Cook the potatoes until fork tender. Drain off the potatoes in a colander.
3. Combine onion, beef, and ¼ cup water in a pan and place the pan over medium heat.
4. As you stir, crumble the meat. Cook until the meat is brown. Stir in peas, potatoes, and a cup of water and cook until peas are cooked.
5. Whisk together 2 tablespoons of broth and cornstarch in a bowl and pour into the pan. Also add remaining broth and stir constantly until thick.
6. Turn off the heat and serve.

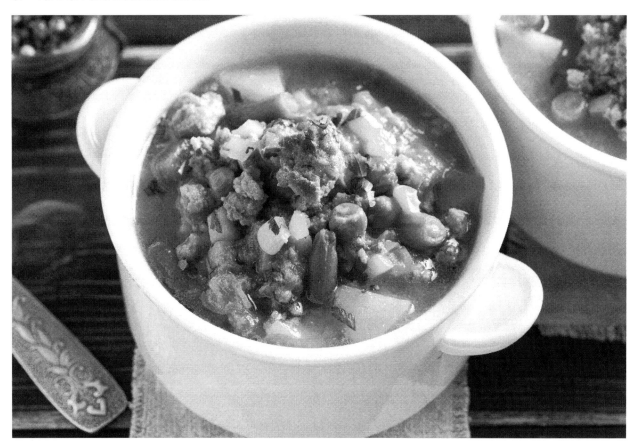

126. BARLEY AND BEEF STEW

Prep. time: 10-12 min | Cooking time: 1 hour and 45-50 min | Servings: 3

INGREDIENTS:

- ½ cup pearl barley, rinsed, soaked in water for an hour, drained
- 1 tablespoon all-purpose flour
- ¼ teaspoon salt
- ¼ cup chopped onion
- 2 small cloves garlic, peeled, sliced
- 1 medium carrot, cut into ¼ inch thick pieces
- ½ teaspoon Mrs. Dash onion herb seasoning

- ½ pound lean beef stew meat, cut into ½ inch chunks
- ⅛ teaspoon pepper
- 1 tablespoon canola oil
- 1 medium stalk celery, chopped
- ½ teaspoon Mrs. Dash onion herb seasoning
- 1 bay leaf
- 4 cups water or more if required

NUTRITIONAL VALUES PER SERVING: 1¼ CUPS	
Calories	246
Fat	8 g
Carbohydrates	21 g
Protein	22 g
Sodium	222 mg
Potassium	369 mg
Phosphorus	175 mg

DIRECTIONS:

1. Add flour and pepper into a bowl and stir.
2. Place meat in a bowl and sprinkle the flour mixture over it and toss until well coated.
3. Pour oil into a pot and heat it over medium heat. Add meat and cook until brown. Remove with a slotted spoon and place on a plate lined with paper towels.
4. Add onion, garlic, and celery into the pot and cook for a couple of minutes.
5. Add water and stir. When it starts boiling, add meat, salt, and bay leaves and stir.
6. Lower the heat. Add barley and stir. Cook covered, on low heat for about 45 minutes. Stir occasionally. Add carrot and herb seasoning and cook for 40-45 minutes or until barley and carrots are cooked. Add more water if required. Ladle into bowls and serve.
7. By reducing the quantity of meat, the protein content in the stew will be further reduced.

127. TURKEY VEGETABLE CHILI

Prep. time: 10 min | Cooking time: 45 min | Servings: 3

INGREDIENTS:

- ½ tablespoon olive oil
- ¼ cup diced onion
- 1 cup cubed zucchini
- 1 teaspoon chili powder
- ¾ teaspoon paprika
- ⅛ teaspoon pepper

- ½ pound lean ground turkey
- 1 clove garlic, minced
- ½ can (from a 14 ounce can) stewed tomatoes, crushed
- ¾ teaspoon ground cumin
- ⅛ teaspoon cayenne pepper

NUTRITIONAL VALUES PER SERVING: ¾ CUP	
Calories	164
Fat	8 g
Carbohydrates	6 g
Protein	17 g
Sodium	214 mg
Potassium	517 mg
Phosphorus	189 mg

DIRECTIONS:

1. Place a pan over medium heat. Spray some cooking spray. Pour oil into the pan.
2. When oil is hot, add turkey, garlic, onion, and zucchini and cook until the vegetables are tender.
3. Discard any extra liquid from the pan. Stir in tomatoes and spices. Cook covered on low heat for about 20 minutes, stirring occasionally.

128. SOUTHERN STYLE STUFFED PEPPERS

Prep. time: 5 min | Cooking time: 1 hour and 10 min | Servings: 2

INGREDIENTS:

- 6 ounces ground beef
- 2 medium bell peppers of any color
- ¾ teaspoon garlic powder
- ½ tablespoon dried parsley
- ¼ cup chopped onion
- 1 cup cooked white rice
- ½ teaspoon black pepper
- 1.5 ounces unsalted tomato sauce

NUTRITIONAL VALUES PER SERVING: 1 BELL PEPPER	
Calories	264
Fat	7 g
Carbohydrates	28 g
Protein	20 g
Sodium	213 mg
Potassium	553 mg
Phosphorus	209 mg

DIRECTIONS:

1. Preheat the oven to 375°F. Grease a baking dish with some cooking spray.
2. Cut off a slice from the top of the bell peppers, near the stem. Remove the seeds and any membranes. Keep them in the baking dish.
3. Cook beef in a pan over medium heat until brown, breaking the meat while stirring.
4. Stir in the rest of the ingredients. Stuff this mixture into the bell peppers.
5. Place the baking dish in the oven and bake for about 50-60 minutes.

129. CHILI CON CARNE

Prep. time: 10 min | Cooking time: 2 hours | Servings: 5

INGREDIENTS:

- ¼ cup diced onion
- ¼ cup diced green bell pepper
- 8 ounces low-sodium stewed tomatoes, blended
- 1 tablespoon chili powder
- ½ stalk celery, chopped
- ¾ pound lean ground beef
- ½ tablespoon canola oil
- ¾ cup water

NUTRITIONAL VALUES PER SERVING: 1 CUP	
Calories	190
Fat	10 g
Carbohydrates	5 g
Protein	20 g
Sodium	116 mg
Potassium	450 mg
Phosphorus	180 mg

DIRECTIONS:

1. Pour oil into a skillet and heat it over medium heat. When oil is hot, add onion, bell pepper, and celery and cook until slightly soft.
2. Stir in the beef and cook until brown. Break the meat as you stir.
3. Add tomatoes, chili powder, and water and stir.
4. Cook covered on low heat for about 2 hours. Stir occasionally.

130. BEEF STROGANOFF

Prep. time: 10 min | Cooking time: 20 min | Servings: 3

INGREDIENTS:

- ½ cup finely chopped onion
- 1 tablespoon low-sodium Worcestershire sauce
- ½ tablespoon mayonnaise—refer to the Vegetarian Reuben sandwich for the recipe
- ½ pound ground beef
- 1 tablespoon flour
- ½ teaspoon pepper
- ⅛ cup sour cream
- 3 ounces wide egg noodles
- ⅛ cup chopped parsley
- 1 small egg, beaten
- ⅛ cup breadcrumbs
- ½ tablespoon unsalted tomato sauce
- 1 ½ tablespoons canola oil
- 1 ½ cups water + extra to cook noodles
- 2 teaspoons low sodium better than bouillon beef
- 1 tablespoon chopped chives
- 1 tablespoon unsalted, chilled butter, cut into cubes
- ½ tablespoon chopped rosemary

NUTRITIONAL VALUES PER SERVING: 1¼ CUPS	
Calories	490
Fat	32 g
Carbohydrates	30 g
Protein	20 g
Sodium	598 mg
Potassium	423 mg
Phosphorus	230 mg

DIRECTIONS:

1. Cook noodles in a pot of water placed over medium heat until al dente. Drain and rinse under cold water. Drain well and set it aside.
2. Combine ¼ teaspoon pepper, onion, egg, Worcestershire sauce, mayonnaise, breadcrumbs, and tomato sauce in a bowl. Add beef and mix well.
3. Make 6 meatballs of the mixture. If you want to make smaller meatballs, make 12 of them.
4. Place a pan over medium heat. Add meatballs and cook until brown all over. Transfer the meatballs onto a plate. Add oil and flour into the pan and mix well.
5. Pour water, beef bouillon, and ¼ teaspoon pepper and mix well. Keep stirring until thick.
6. Remove the pan from heat. Add chives and sour cream and stir. Cover and set it aside.
7. Place another pan over medium heat. Add pasta, butter, and a sprinkle of water and mix well. Add parsley and rosemary and mix well. Heat thoroughly.
8. Divide the noodles into 3 bowls. Divide the meatballs among the bowls.
9. Divide the sauce and pour over the meatballs and noodles.

131. TURKEY SLOPPY JOES

Prep. time: 5-8 min | Cooking time: 20 min | Servings: 3

INGREDIENTS:

- ¼ cup diced red onion
- ¾ pound ground turkey (7% fat)
- 1 tablespoon brown sugar
- ½ cup low-sodium tomato sauce
- 3 hamburger buns
- ¼ cup diced green bell pepper
- ½ tablespoon Mrs. Dash Chicken grilling blend seasoning
- ½ tablespoon low-sodium Worcestershire sauce

NUTRITIONAL VALUES PER SERVING: 1 BELL PEPPER	
Calories	290
Fat	9 g
Carbohydrates	28 g
Protein	24 g
Sodium	288 mg
Potassium	513 mg
Phosphorus	237 mg

DIRECTIONS:

1. Add turkey, onion, and bell pepper into a skillet. Place the skillet over medium-high heat and cook the turkey mixture.
2. Combine sugar, seasoning, tomato sauce, and Worcestershire sauce in a bowl.
3. Pour this mixture into the skillet once the turkey is cooked.
4. Lower the heat and simmer for about 7-8 minutes. Turn off the heat.
5. Split the hamburger buns. Place the turkey mixture on the bottom half of the buns. Cover with the top half of the buns and serve.

132. TURKEY BREAST WITH CARROTS AND CRANBERRY GRAVY

Prep. time: 10 min | Cooking time: 50-60 hours | Servings: 3

INGREDIENTS:

- ⅛ cup chopped onion
- 1 cup sliced carrots
- ½ cup cranberry sauce
- 3 tablespoons sliced celery
- 9 ounces boneless, skinless turkey breast
- ¼ teaspoon chicken bouillon granules
- ½ teaspoon poultry seasoning, unsalted

NUTRITIONAL VALUES PER SERVING: 2½ ounces turkey with ⅓ cup vegetables and ¼ cup cranberry gravy	
Calories	216
Fat	6 g
Carbohydrates	25 g
Protein	18 g
Sodium	183 mg
Potassium	373 mg
Phosphorus	187 mg

DIRECTIONS:

1. Place turkey and vegetables in a Dutch oven. Add poultry seasoning and bouillon granules and stir.
2. Add cranberry sauce and mix well. Cover the pot and cook on low heat for about an hour or until meat is tender. You can also cook it in a slow cooker if you have one. In the slow cooker, add all the ingredients into the slow cooker and cook on High for 2-3 hours.
3. Take out the turkey from the pot and place on your cutting board. Let it rest for about 10 minutes. Cut into slices and divide into 3 plates.
4. Divide the vegetables and cranberry gravy equally and pour over the turkey. Serve.

133. CURRIED TURKEY AND RICE

Prep. time: 5 min | Cooking time: 10-12 min | Servings: 3

INGREDIENTS:

- ½ teaspoon vegetable oil
- ½ medium onion, chopped
- 1 teaspoon curry powder
- ½ teaspoon sugar
- 1 tablespoon flour
- ¼ cup non-dairy creamer
- 1 cup cooked white rice
- ½ pound turkey breast, cut into 3 cutlets
- ½ tablespoon unsalted margarine
- ½ cup low-sodium chicken broth

NUTRITIONAL VALUES PER SERVING: 1 BURGER	
Calories	154
Fat	5 g
Carbohydrates	20 g
Protein	8 g
Sodium	27 mg
Potassium	156 mg
Phosphorus	88 mg

DIRECTIONS:

1. Pour oil into a skillet and let it heat over medium heat. Add turkey and cook until it is not pink anymore. Remove turkey onto a plate. Cover loosely with aluminum foil.
2. Add margarine into the skillet. Once margarine melts, add onion and cook for a couple of minutes. Add curry powder and sauté for 2-3 minutes.
3. Stir in the flour. Stir constantly for a minute. Add broth, sugar, and creamer, stirring constantly. Keep stirring until thick. Add turkey and mix well. Heat thoroughly.
4. Place ⅓ cup rice on each of 3 plates. Place 1 cutlet on each plate, over the rice. Divide the gravy and spoon over the cutlets. Serve immediately.

134. TURKEY MEATBALL SKEWERS

Prep. time: 15 min | Cooking time: 12 min | Servings: 4

INGREDIENTS:

- ½ pound lean ground turkey (7% fat)
- 1 small egg
- ½ teaspoon Mrs. Dash salt-free seasoning
- ½ teaspoon dried basil
- ½ large bell pepper, cut into 1 inch squares
- ¼ cup plain panko breadcrumbs
- ¼ large onion, cut into 1 inch squares
- ¼ large onion, minced
- ½ teaspoon garlic powder
- ½ large zucchini, cut into 1 inch cubes

NUTRITIONAL VALUES PER SERVING: 1 skewer with 3-5 vegetable pieces, without serving	
Calories	178
Fat	8 g
Carbohydrates	10 g
Protein	18 g
Sodium	113 mg
Potassium	381 mg
Phosphorus	197 mg

DIRECTIONS:

1. Place turkey, egg, panko, minced onion, garlic powder, and Mrs. Dash seasoning in a bowl and mix well. Make 12 equal portions of the mixture and shape into balls.
2. If you are using wooden skewers, soak them in water for 30 minutes before grilling.
3. Set up your grill and preheat it to medium heat.
4. Build the skewers by threading 3 meatballs on each skewer, alternating with bell pepper, onion, and zucchini. Make sure to divide the vegetables equally. Grill on medium heat for 10-12 mins.
5. You can serve the skewers with rice or with a salad.

135. BAKED PORK CHOPS

Prep. time: 10 min | Cooking time: 50 min + chilling time | Servings: 3

INGREDIENTS:

- ¼ cup all-purpose flour
- ⅛ cup water
- 3 center-cut pork chops (3.5 ounces each)
- ½ teaspoon paprika
- 3 canned peach halves
- 1 small egg
- 6 tablespoons crumbled corn flakes
- 1 tablespoon unsalted margarine
- ⅛ teaspoon salt

NUTRITIONAL VALUES PER SERVING	
Calories	282
Fat	10 g
Carbohydrates	25 g
Protein	23 g
Sodium	263 mg
Potassium	394 mg
Phosphorus	203 mg

DIRECTIONS:

1. Place flour on a plate. Place cornflakes on another plate.
2. Whisk together water and egg in a bowl.
3. First, coat the pork chops in flour. Next, dunk in egg. Shake off excess egg and roll the pork chops in cornflakes and place on the baking sheet. Pour melted margarine over the pork chops. Sprinkle salt and paprika on top. Chill for 1-4 hours.
4. Preheat the oven to 375°F. Grease a baking sheet with some cooking spray.
5. Place the baking sheet in the oven and bake for 40 minutes or until the internal temperature in the center of the meat shows 145°F on the meat thermometer.
6. Remove the pork chops from the oven and let it sit for 3-5 minutes before serving.
7. Place the peach halves on the baking sheet during the last 15 minutes of baking. You can cook the pork chops and peach halves on a preheated grill as well.

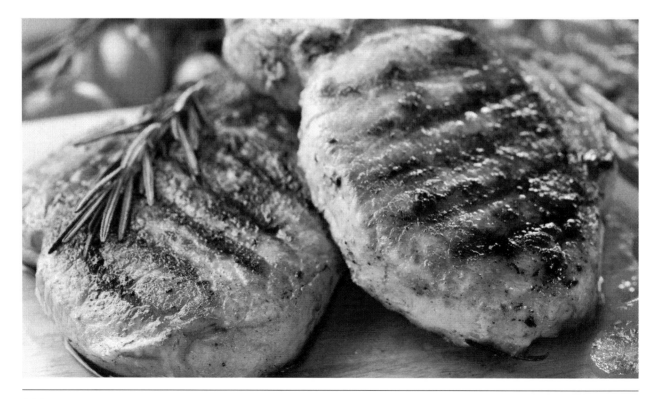

136. PORK CHOPS WITH CRANBERRY SAUCE

Prep. time: 5 min | Cooking time: 15-18 min | Servings: 3

INGREDIENTS:

- 3 boneless pork loin chops (4 ounces each)
- 1 teaspoon cornstarch
- 1 teaspoon honey
- ½ tablespoon minced parsley
- ½ tablespoon minced tarragon
- Coarsely ground pepper to taste
- ½ cup cran-apple juice
- 6 tablespoons dried, sweetened cranberries
- 1 ½ cups cooked white rice

NUTRITIONAL VALUES PER SERVING: 1 PORK CHOP WITH ½ CUP RICE	
Calories	397
Fat	13 g
Carbohydrates	45 g
Protein	25 g
Sodium	76 mg
Potassium	410 mg
Phosphorus	267 mg

DIRECTIONS:

1. Spray a nonstick skillet with some cooking spray. Place the skillet over medium heat.
2. Season the pork chops with pepper and place in the pan. Cook for 3-4 minutes, until the underside is light brown. Turn the pork chops over and cook the other side for 3-4 minutes until light brown. Transfer the chops onto a plate and keep it warm.
3. Meanwhile, whisk together honey, cornstarch, and cran-apple juice in a bowl. Add cranberries and herbs and stir. Pour the mixture into the skillet and stir constantly until thick.
4. Add the pork chops into the pan and stir well. Lower the heat and cook covered for 4-6 minutes or until the internal temperature of the meat in the thickest part shows 160°F.

137. MARINATED SHRIMP

Prep. time: 10 min + marinating time | Cooking time: 0 min | Servings: 3

INGREDIENTS:

- 10 ounces large shrimp
- 3 tablespoons vinegar
- ¼ teaspoon salt
- ½ teaspoon celery seeds
- ½ small cloves garlic, peeled, minced
- ½ cup thinly sliced onions
- 6 tablespoons oil
- 1 teaspoon capers along with a little of canned liquid
- ¼ teaspoon whole cloves
- A dash red pepper sauce
- 2 bay leaves

NUTRITIONAL VALUES PER SERVING: 6 SHRIMP	
Calories	188
Fat	12 g
Carbohydrates	2.4 g
Protein	17 g
Sodium	180 mg
Potassium	187 mg
Phosphorus	162 mg

DIRECTIONS:

1. Place shrimp in a baking dish. Scatter onions over it. Place bay leaves on top.
2. Add vinegar, salt, celery seeds, garlic, oil, cloves, red pepper sauce and capers into a bowl and whisk well. Pour over the shrimp and onions.
3. Chill for at least 24 hours.
4. Serve chilled.

138. SPICY PORK CHOPS WITH APPLES

Prep. time: 5 min | Cooking time: 35 min | Servings: 3

INGREDIENTS:

- 1 clove garlic, peeled, minced
- ½ teaspoon ground ginger
- ⅛ teaspoon pepper
- ¼ teaspoon + ⅛ teaspoon salt
- ¼ teaspoon sugar
- ⅛ teaspoon ground cumin
- 3 large pork chops
- 1 medium apple, cored, cut into 1 inch thick slices
- 1 medium onion, cut into ¾ inch thick wedges

NUTRITIONAL VALUES PER SERVING: 1 pork chop with ⅓ apple and ⅓ onion	
Calories	215
Fat	13 g
Carbohydrates	9.8 g
Protein	15 g
Sodium	330 mg
Potassium	288 mg
Phosphorus	126 mg

DIRECTIONS:

1. Preheat the oven to 375°F.
2. Add all the spices, sugar and salt into a bowl and stir.
3. Rub the spice blend all over the pork chops and place in a small, glass baking dish.
4. Place apple slices and onion slices in between the pork pieces.
5. Crumple some foil and place all around the inner sides of the dish so that the ingredients are close together. They should not fall apart. Cover the dish with another sheet of foil.
6. Place the baking dish in the oven and bake for about 30-35 minutes.
7. Remove the foil on the top as well as the ones inside the dish and separate the apples, onion, and pork chops. Bake for another 15 minutes or until light brown on top.
8. Place a pork chop on each plate. Divide the apple and onion slices among the plates and serve over rice if desired.

139. BAKED FISH À LA MUSHROOMS

NUTRITIONAL VALUES PER SERVING	
Calories	155
Fat	7 g
Carbohydrates	2 g
Protein	21 g
Sodium	110 mg
Potassium	561 mg
Phosphorus	225 mg

Prep. time: 5 min | Cooking time: 20 min | Servings: 2

INGREDIENTS:

- ½ pound fresh cod fillets
- ⅛ cup chopped white onion
- ¾ cup sliced fresh mushrooms
- ½ teaspoon dried thyme, crushed
- 1 tablespoon unsalted margarine

DIRECTIONS:

1. Preheat the oven to 450°F. Grease a baking dish with some cooking spray and keep the fish fillets in the dish.
2. Add margarine into a pan and place the pan over medium heat. Once it melts, add onion and mushroom and cook until the vegetables are tender.
3. Turn off the heat and spread the vegetables over the fish. Sprinkle thyme over the vegetables.
4. Place the baking dish in the oven and set the timer for 12-15 minutes, until the fish cooks through.

140. CARIBBEAN-STYLE COCONUT FISH STEW

Prep. time: 15 min | Cooking time: 25 min | Servings: 2

INGREDIENTS:

- A handful chopped cilantro + extra to garnish
- ¼ habanero pepper or ½ Serrano pepper, deseeded
- ¼ teaspoon annatto seeds
- ½ medium onion, sliced divided
- 1 tablespoon olive oil
- ¼ small yellow bell pepper, thinly sliced
- Juice of ½ lime
- ¼ small red bell pepper, thinly sliced
- 4 ounces cod, cut into 2 inch pieces
- 1 clove garlic, sliced
- ½ teaspoon smoked paprika
- A pinch sea salt
- ½ can (from a 14.1 ounce can) coconut milk
- ½ cup water

NUTRITIONAL VALUES PER SERVING: 1 CUP	
Calories	300
Fat	25 g
Carbohydrates	11 g
Protein	12 g
Sodium	202 mg
Potassium	555 mg
Phosphorus	185 mg

DIRECTIONS:

1. Place cilantro, habanero pepper, annatto seeds, half the onion, garlic, paprika, salt, and a tablespoon of coconut milk in a blender. Blend until you get a paste.
2. Pour oil into a saucepan and place the saucepan over medium-high heat. When oil is hot, add onion and bell peppers and cook until the vegetables are slightly tender.
3. Add water and remaining coconut milk. Add the blended paste as well. Mix well.
4. When the mixture starts boiling, lower the heat and simmer for about 8-10 minutes.
5. Stir in fish. Cook covered for about 5 minutes.
6. Add lime juice and mix well. Sprinkle cilantro on top and serve.

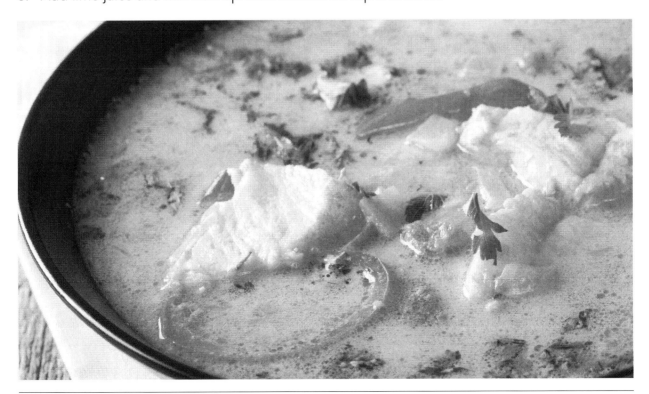

141. SEAFOOD GUMBO

Prep. time: 10 min | Cooking time: 30-35 min | Servings: 6

INGREDIENTS:

- ¼ cup + ½ tablespoon canola oil, divided
- ½ yellow onion, chopped
- ½ tablespoon salt-free Cajun seasoning
- 4 ounces lean smoked turkey sausage, sliced
- 3 ounces canned crab
- ¼ pound cooked shrimp
- 1 skinless chicken breast, chopped
- 1 ½ cups chopped frozen okra
- 1 ½ stalks celery, chopped
- ½ red bell pepper, chopped
- ¼ cup flour
- 4 cups low-sodium chicken broth

NUTRITIONAL VALUES PER SERVING: 1 CUP	
Calories	240
Fat	2 g
Carbohydrates	19 g
Protein	10 g
Sodium	320 mg
Potassium	425 mg
Phosphorus	156 mg

DIRECTIONS:

1. Pour ½ tablespoon canola oil into a soup pot and place the pot over medium heat.
2. Once oil is hot, add onion, celery, bell pepper, turkey sausage, and chicken and sauté for about 8-10 minutes. Transfer the chicken mixture into a bowl.
3. Pour ¼ cup oil into the pot. Add flour and keep stirring until roux is formed.
4. Add Cajun seasoning and mix well for about 30-60 minutes, depending on how toasted you prefer the spices. Pour chicken broth in a thin stream, stirring all the time while adding the broth.
5. Raise the heat to medium-high heat and let the mixture cook until slightly thick.
6. Lower the heat to medium heat and stir in crab, shrimp, the chicken mixture, and okra.
7. Heat thoroughly. Serve hot.

142. CUCUMBER SALAD

Prep. time: 10 min | Cooking time: 10 min + chilling time | Servings: 4

INGREDIENTS:

- 2 medium cucumbers, peel if desired, sliced
- ¼ cup sugar
- ¼ cup water
- 1 sprig dill (optional)
- ½ medium onion, sliced
- ½ cup white vinegar
- ⅛ teaspoon salt

NUTRITIONAL VALUES PER SERVING: 1 CUP	
Calories	28
Fat	0.2 g
Carbohydrates	4.6 g
Protein	0.8 g
Sodium	77.3 mg
Potassium	191.8 mg
Phosphorus	30 mg

DIRECTIONS:

1. Place cucumbers and onion in a bowl and toss well. Add salt and dill and mix well.
2. Combine water, sugar, and vinegar in a saucepan. Place the saucepan over medium heat and stir until sugar dissolves completely and the solution is hot.
3. Turn off the heat and pour into the bowl of cucumbers. Stir well.
4. Let it rest for 30 minutes.
5. Serve.

143. EGGPLANT SEAFOOD CASSEROLE

Prep. time: 15 min | Cooking time: 45 min | Servings: 4

INGREDIENTS:

- 1 medium eggplant, cut into 1 inch cubes
- ½ bell pepper, chopped
- 1 clove garlic, chopped
- ½ medium onion, chopped
- ¼ cup chopped celery
- ⅛ cup olive oil
- ½ tablespoon Worcestershire sauce
- ¼ teaspoon Tabasco sauce
- ⅛ cup grated parmesan

- cheese
- 2 medium eggs
- ¼ pound boiled shrimp
- ½ pound lump crab meat
- 1 tablespoon unsalted butter, melted
- ⅛ cup lemon juice
- ⅛ teaspoon creole seasoning
- 3 tablespoons uncooked rice
- A pinch cayenne pepper
- ¼ cup breadcrumbs

NUTRITIONAL VALUES PER SERVING: 1 CUP	
Calories	216
Fat	12 g
Carbohydrates	14 g
Protein	13 g
Sodium	229 mg
Potassium	359 mg
Phosphorus	148 mg

DIRECTIONS:

1. Preheat the oven to 350°F. Grease a casserole dish with some cooking spray and keep the fish fillets in the dish.
2. Cook eggplant in a pot of water until tender. Drain in a colander and keep it in a bowl.
3. Pour oil into a pan and let it heat over medium heat. Add onion, garlic, celery, and bell pepper and cook until the vegetables are tender.
4. Transfer the vegetables into the bowl of eggplant. Add eggs, cayenne pepper, cheese, rice, Tabasco, lemon juice, creole seasoning, and Worcestershire sauce and mix well.
5. Add crab and shrimp and fold in gently. Scoop the mixture into the casserole dish.
6. Combine breadcrumbs and butter in a bowl and scatter over the casserole.
7. Place the casserole dish in the oven and set the timer for 25-30 minutes or until brown on top.

144. CREAMY TUNA MACARONI

Prep. time: 5 min | Cooking time: 0 min + chilling time | Servings: 2

INGREDIENTS:

- 6 tablespoons mayonnaise
- ¾ cup cooked shell macaroni
- ¼ cup cooked peas
- ½ tablespoon dried dill weed
- 1 tablespoon vinegar

- ½ can (from a 6 ½ ounce can) tuna, unsalted or water packed, drained
- ¼ cup chopped celery

NUTRITIONAL VALUES PER SERVING: 1 CUP	
Calories	421
Fat	31 g
Carbohydrates	20 g
Protein	15 g
Sodium	379 mg
Potassium	204 mg
Phosphorus	122 mg

DIRECTIONS:

1. Place peas, dill, vinegar, celery, and mayonnaise in a bowl. Stir until well combined.
2. Add tuna and macaroni and stir. Cover the bowl and chill until use.

145. SEAFOOD CORN CHOWDER

Prep. time: 10 min | Cooking time: 10-12 min | Servings: 5

INGREDIENTS:

- ½ tablespoon unsalted butter
- 3 tablespoons chopped celery
- ¼ cup chopped red bell pepper
- ¼ cup chopped green bell pepper
- ½ cup chopped onion
- ½ tablespoon all-purpose white flour
- 1 cup liquid nondairy creamer
- 5 ounces surimi imitation crab chunks
- ¼ teaspoon pepper
- 7 ounces low-sodium chicken broth
- 3 ounces evaporated milk
- 1 cup frozen corn kernels
- ¼ teaspoon paprika

NUTRITIONAL VALUES PER SERVING: 1 CUP	
Calories	173
Fat	7 g
Carbohydrates	22 g
Protein	8 g
Sodium	160 mg
Potassium	258 mg
Phosphorus	181 mg

DIRECTIONS:

1. Add butter into a soup pot and place the pot over medium heat. Once butter melts, add onion, bell peppers, and celery and cook until tender.
2. Stir in the flour. Keep stirring for a couple of minutes.
3. Add broth, stirring constantly. Keep stirring until slightly thick.
4. Add spices, non dairy creamer, corn, crab, and evaporated milk and stir. Heat thoroughly but not boiling. Ladle into bowls and serve.

146. SAUTÉED MUNG BEANS (MUNGGO GUISADO)

Prep. time: 10 min | Cooking time: 30 min | Servings: 4

INGREDIENTS:

- ½ cup thinly sliced lean pork (2 ounces)
- ½ tablespoon corn oil
- ½ cup chopped white onion
- ½ teaspoon pepper
- ½ cup frozen spinach
- ½ tablespoon minced garlic
- ½ cup chopped tomatoes
- 2 cups water
- ½ teaspoon salt
- ½ cup peeled, deveined shrimp
- 1 ¾ cups pre cooked mung beans

NUTRITIONAL VALUES PER SERVING: 1 CUP	
Calories	160
Fat	4 g
Carbohydrates	19 g
Protein	13 g
Sodium	350 mg
Potassium	370 mg
Phosphorus	223 mg

DIRECTIONS:

1. Pour oil into a skillet and heat it over medium heat. When oil is hot, add garlic and cook until light brown.
2. Stir in tomatoes and onion and cook until the tomatoes have a bit of crinkly skin.
3. Stir in pork and cook until light brown. Pour water and cook for 12-13 minutes on low heat.
4. Add mung beans, salt, and pepper and cook for another 12 -13 minutes.
5. Stir in shrimp and spinach and cook until shrimp turn pink.

147. SHRIMP AND PASTA SALAD

Prep. time: 15 min | Cooking time: 0 min + chilling time | Servings: 5

INGREDIENTS:

SALAD:
- 6 ounces uncooked tri-color pasta
- ¼ large yellow bell pepper, diced
- ¼ large red bell pepper, diced
- ¼ red onion, diced
- 8-10 baby carrots, cut into thick round slices
- ¼ English cucumber, peeled, cubed
- 2 stalks celery, diced

- ¾ cup cauliflower florets (about ¾ inch)
- ¼ pound cooked shrimp

DRESSING:
- 2 tablespoons balsamic vinegar
- ½ tablespoon Dijon mustard
- 6 tablespoons olive oil
- 2 tablespoons honey
- ¼ teaspoon black pepper
- ¼ teaspoon garlic powder

NUTRITIONAL VALUES PER SERVING: ⅕ RECIPE	
Calories	473
Fat	4 g
Carbohydrates	65 g
Protein	16 g
Sodium	143 mg
Potassium	312 mg
Phosphorus	117 mg

DIRECTIONS:

1. Cook pasta in a pot of water until al dente. Drain in a colander and rinse well under cold running water.
2. Whisk together all the dressing ingredients except oil in a bowl. Pour oil in a thin drizzle, whisking constantly while adding the oil.
3. Combine shrimp, pasta, and vegetables in a bowl. Drizzle the dressing over the salad. Toss well.
4. Cover the bowl and chill for 5-8 hours.

148. GLAZED CARROTS

Prep. time: 10 min | Cooking time: 25 min | Servings: 3-4

INGREDIENTS:

- ½ pound carrots, peeled
- 2 tablespoons brown sugar
- ½ tablespoon unsalted butter
- A pinch pepper

NUTRITIONAL VALUES PER SERVING: ½ CUP	
Calories	124
Fat	3.2 g
Carbohydrates	24.4 g
Protein	1.1 g
Sodium	82.5 mg
Potassium	383 mg
Phosphorus	41.2 mg

DIRECTIONS:

1. Pour enough water into a pot such that it is about 2 inches in height from the bottom of the pot. Place the pot over high heat and let it start boiling.
2. Place carrots in a steamer basket and place the basket in the pot. Cover the steamer basket and cook for 10 minutes or until fork tender.
3. To make glaze: Combine butter and sugar in a small pan. Place the pan over medium heat and stir often until sugar melts. Turn off the heat.
4. Place carrots in a bowl. Pour the butter mixture over the carrots and toss well.
5. Serve.

149. FRESH TOFU SPRING ROLLS

Prep. time: 15 min | Cooking time: 15 min + chilling time | Servings: 3

INGREDIENTS:

- 6 Romaine lettuce leaves, halved lengthwise
- 1 medium carrot, peeled, cut into matchsticks
- 8 ounces firm tofu, drained, dried with paper towels, cut into 6 long pieces
- 1 small red onion, thinly sliced
- ¾ teaspoon granulated garlic
- ¼ teaspoon pepper
- 6 rice wrappers
- ¾ teaspoon ground cumin
- ⅛ teaspoon sea salt
- ½ tablespoon olive oil

NUTRITIONAL VALUES PER SERVING: 2 SPRING ROLLS (WITHOUT DRESSING OR DIP)

Calories	156
Fat	5 g
Carbohydrates	20 g
Protein	8 g
Sodium	161 mg
Potassium	302 mg
Phosphorus	93 mg

DIRECTIONS:

1. Boil a pot of water. Turn off the heat and cover the pot.
2. Combine cumin, salt, garlic, and pepper in a bowl and sprinkle it on top of the tofu slices.
3. Pour oil into a nonstick pan and place the pan over medium heat. When oil is hot, add tofu strips into the pan but place it with the seasoned side touching the bottom of the pan. Cook until the underside is light brown.
4. Turn the tofu strips over and cook the other side until light brown. Turn off the heat. Transfer the tofu onto a plate.
5. While the tofu is cooling, pour the boiled water into a bowl, which should be wide enough to dip a rice wrapper.
6. Place a rice wrapper in the bowl of hot water. In a minute or so, the wrapper will become soft. Carefully lift it and keep it on a plate. Place another wrapper in the bowl of water to soften.
7. Keep 2 lettuce halves in the middle of the softened wrapper (which is on the plate). Scatter ⅙ of each—carrot, onion and tofu over the lettuce. Fold like a burrito and place on a plate.
8. Repeat steps 6-7 and make the remaining spring rolls. Cover the plate with cling wrap and chill for a few hours.
9. Serve it chilled with any low-sodium dressing or dip of your choice.

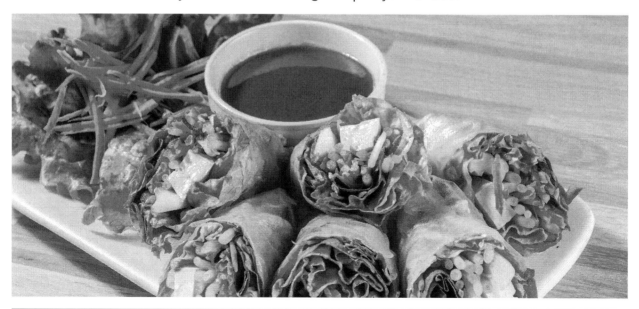

150. VEGGIE BURGER

Prep. time: 20 min | Cooking time: 10 min | Servings: 4

INGREDIENTS:

- 1 cup chopped mushrooms
- ½ cup minced broccoli
- 2 small eggs, beaten
- ½ can (from a 15 ounces can) low-sodium black beans, drained, rinsed
- ¼ cup minced red onion
- 1 slice stale white bread
- ¼ teaspoon pepper
- ½ teaspoon garlic powder
- ½ teaspoon Worcestershire sauce
- 1 tablespoon olive oil
- ⅛ cup shredded parmesan cheese

NUTRITIONAL VALUES
PER SERVING: 1 BURGER
(WITHOUT SERVING OPTIONS)

Calories	155
Fat	7 g
Carbohydrates	16 g
Protein	8 g
Sodium	114 mg
Potassium	277 mg
Phosphorus	139 mg

DIRECTIONS:

1. Tear up the bread slice and place in a small blender. Blend until you get breadcrumbs.
2. Place black beans in a bowl and mash with a fork until most of it is mashed and only a few chunks of the beans are remaining.
3. Stir in breadcrumbs, broccoli, mushrooms, eggs, pepper, cheese, Worcestershire sauce, garlic powder, and onion. Make 4 equal portions of the mixture and shape into patties.
4. Pour oil into a skillet and heat it over medium heat. When oil is hot, add patties and cook until the underside is golden brown. Turn the patties over and cook the other side until golden brown.
5. Serve burgers over hamburger buns, lettuce leaves, or over wraps with renal diet friendly toppings of your choice.

151. CARROT AND PARSNIP SOUP

Prep. time: 10 min | Cooking time: 25-30 min | Servings: 3

INGREDIENTS:

- 1 ½ tablespoons olive oil
- 1 teaspoon paprika
- ¼ teaspoon chili powder
- ⅛ teaspoon pepper
- ½ teaspoon garlic powder
- A tiny pinch sea salt
- 1 cup sliced parsnip
- ¼ cup thinly sliced celery
- 1 cup sliced carrots
- ½ tablespoon chopped chives
- Juice of ½ lime
- 2 cups low-sodium vegetable broth
- 1 tablespoon unsalted pumpkin seeds

NUTRITIONAL VALUES
PER SERVING: 1 BOWL

Calories	143
Fat	8 g
Carbohydrates	16 g
Protein	2 g
Sodium	169 mg
Potassium	198 mg
Phosphorus	91 mg

DIRECTIONS:

1. Pour oil into a soup pot and place the pot over medium heat. When oil is hot, add celery, salt, and spices and cook until slightly tender, stirring occasionally.
2. Stir in parsnip and carrot and mix well. Cook for a couple of minutes.
3. Pour in the broth. Cover the pot with a lid, only partial covering. Cook on low heat until the vegetables are cooked. Blend the soup until smooth. Divide the soup equally into 3 soup bowls.
4. Sprinkle pumpkin seeds and chives on top. Drizzle lime juice and serve.

152. SPRING VEGETABLE SOUP

Prep. time: 10 min | Cooking time: 60 min | Servings: 10

INGREDIENTS:

- 2 cups stringed, fresh green beans pieces (2 inch pieces)
- 1 cup chopped onions
- 1 cup chopped carrot
- 1 cup frozen corn
- 1 ½ cups chopped celery
- 1 cup chopped mushrooms
- 2 teaspoons garlic powder
- 4 tablespoons olive oil
- 2 teaspoons dried oregano
- ½ teaspoon salt
- 2 medium Roma tomatoes, chopped
- 8 cups low-sodium vegetable broth

NUTRITIONAL VALUES PER SERVING: 1 CUP	
Calories	114
Fat	6 g
Carbohydrates	13 g
Protein	2 g
Sodium	262 mg
Potassium	400 mg
Phosphorus	108 mg

DIRECTIONS:

1. Pour oil into a soup pot and heat it over medium heat. When oil is hot, add onion and celery and cook for a few minutes until slightly soft.
2. Stir in carrots, corn, celery, mushrooms, tomatoes, broth, garlic powder, oregano, and tomatoes and mix well.
3. When the mixture starts boiling, lower the heat and cook for about 45-50 minutes.

153. THAI RED CURRY VEGETABLES AND RICE

Prep. time: 10 min | Cooking time: 20-25 min | Servings: 2

INGREDIENTS:

- ½ small shallot, chopped
- ½ cup green beans pieces (1 inch pieces)
- 1 cup cauliflower florets (1 inch florets)
- 1 medium carrot, cut into 1 inch pieces
- ½ tablespoon canola oil
- ½ cup plain coconut milk
- ½ kaffir lime leaf
- Juice of ½ lime
- 1 tablespoon Thai red curry paste, unsalted
- 7 ounces low-sodium vegetable broth
- 1 cup cooked white rice

NUTRITIONAL VALUES PER SERVING: ½ cup rice with 1 ½ cups vegetable curry	
Calories	210
Fat	17 g
Carbohydrates	26 g
Protein	8 g
Sodium	277 mg
Potassium	588 mg
Phosphorus	142 mg

DIRECTIONS:

1. Pour oil into a pan and heat it over medium heat. When oil is hot, add shallot and cook until soft.
2. Stir in red curry paste; keep stirring for a few seconds until you get a nice aroma.
3. Pour broth and coconut milk. Add lime leaf and mix well.
4. Cover the pan and let the mixture start simmering.
5. Add the vegetables and cover the pan once again. Simmer until fork tender.
6. Remove the pot from heat. Discard the lime leaf. Add lime juice and stir.
7. Serve rice with vegetable curry.

154. SPAGHETTI AND ASPARAGUS CARBONARA

Prep. time: 10 min | Cooking time: 10 min | Servings: 3

INGREDIENTS:

- 1 teaspoon canola oil
- 1 small egg, beaten
- 2 tablespoons low-sodium chicken stock
- 1 cup fresh asparagus pieces (1 inch pieces)
- ¼ cup chopped scallions
- 1 ½ tablespoons shredded parmesan cheese
- ½ cup diced onions
- ½ cup heavy cream
- 1 ½ cups cooked spiral noodle pasta
- ½ teaspoon freshly cracked black pepper
- 1 ½ tablespoons meatless bacon bits

NUTRITIONAL VALUES PER SERVING: 1 BURGER (WITHOUT SERVING OPTIONS)	
Calories	304
Fat	19 g
Carbohydrates	27 g
Protein	9 g
Sodium	141 mg
Potassium	287 mg
Phosphorus	143 mg

DIRECTIONS:

1. Pour oil into a nonstick pan and heat over medium-high heat. When the oil is hot, add onion and cook until light brown. Reduce to medium heat.
2. Add egg and cream into a bowl and whisk well. Pour the egg mixture into the pan and keep stirring until the egg begins to set.
3. Stir in asparagus, stock, pepper, and pasta. Heat thoroughly, stirring constantly. Remove from heat.
4. Divide into 3 plates. Divide the scallions, cheese, and bacon equally and sprinkle over the pasta.
5. Serve hot.

---

155. HOLUSHKI NOODLES AND CABBAGE

Prep. time: 10 min | Cooking time: 1 hour and 15 min | Servings: 3-4

NUTRITIONAL VALUES PER SERVING: 1 CUP	
Calories	167
Fat	6 g
Carbohydrates	23 g
Protein	5 g
Sodium	75 mg
Potassium	263 mg
Phosphorus	67 mg

INGREDIENTS:

- 4 cups shredded cabbage
- 3 tablespoons water
- 3 tablespoons margarine
- ⅛ teaspoon pepper
- 1 medium white onion, chopped
- 4 ounces kluski noodles, uncooked

DIRECTIONS:

1. Combine onion, water, and cabbage in a pan. Cook over medium-low heat for about 40 minutes until tender. Stir often. Sprinkle some water whenever required to prevent burning.
2. Cook the noodles following the directions given on the package of noodles, but do not add salt while cooking. Drain and keep it aside.
3. Once cabbage is cooked, make sure to dry up the water. Stir in margarine and cook for another 10-12 minutes.
4. Add pepper and noodles and mix well. Heat thoroughly and serve.

156. SINGAPORE RICE NOODLES

Prep. time: 10 min | Cooking time: 45 min | Servings: 3

INGREDIENTS:

- 4 ounces thin rice noodles
- 1 medium carrot, cut into matchsticks
- ½ cup sliced snow peas (slice it on the bias)
- 2 scallions, thinly sliced
- 7 ounces low-sodium chicken broth
- ½ tablespoon curry powder
- ½ tablespoon canola oil
- ½ bunch cilantro, thinly sliced
- ½ tablespoon low-sodium soy sauce
- ¼ teaspoon garlic powder
- 1 large egg, beaten

NUTRITIONAL VALUES PER SERVING: 1 BOWL	
Calories	226
Fat	6 g
Carbohydrates	30 g
Protein	12 g
Sodium	216 mg
Potassium	350 mg
Phosphorus	194 mg

DIRECTIONS:

1. Cook the rice noodles following the instructions on the package. Drain the noodles and keep it in a bowl.
2. Whisk together broth, curry powder, soy sauce, oil, and garlic powder in a pan. When the mixture starts boiling, stir in the carrots, and snow peas. Cook for some time until the carrots are tender. Remove the pan from heat.
3. Mix in noodles and half the cilantro. Cover the pan and keep it aside.
4. Place another pan over medium heat. Spray some cooking spray. Add egg into the pan and stir often until eggs are cooked. If there are large pieces of egg, break into smaller pieces.
5. Combine the eggs with the noodle mixture.
6. Divide equally into 3 bowls. Top with scallions and remaining cilantro and serve.

157. ZUCCHINI CASSEROLE

Prep. time: 25 min | Cooking time: 45 min | Servings: 2

INGREDIENTS:

- 1 large egg
- 1 tablespoon chopped onion
- ¼ teaspoon Mrs. Dash herb seasoning blend
- ½ medium zucchini, trimmed, chopped
- 1 ½ slices white bread, cubed
- ¼ cup liquid nondairy creamer
- A pinch salt
- ⅛ teaspoon pepper
- 1.5 ounces cream cheese, cubed

NUTRITIONAL VALUES PER SERVING: ¾ CUP	
Calories	216
Fat	14 g
Carbohydrates	16 g
Protein	7 g
Sodium	318 mg
Potassium	232 mg
Phosphorus	123 mg

DIRECTIONS:

1. Preheat the oven to 325°F. Prepare a small casserole dish by greasing it with some cooking spray.
2. Crack egg into a bowl. Add onion, pepper, non dairy creamer, salt, and Mrs. Dash seasoning. And stir until well-combined.
3. Stir in the cream cheese, zucchini, and bread. Let it rest for 10 minutes.
4. Spoon the mixture into the prepared casserole dish. Place the baking dish in the oven and bake for about 40 minutes or until light brown on top.

158. CRISPY LENTIL AND COLLARD GREEN SALAD

Prep. time: 10 min | Cooking time: 10 min | Servings: 1

INGREDIENTS:

- ½ teaspoon sunflower oil
- Pepper to taste
- ¼ jalapeño, diced, deseed if desired
- ½ teaspoon ground mustard seeds
- ⅛ teaspoon sea salt
- 1 tablespoon minced mint leaves
- 1 tablespoon lime juice
- 1 small mandarin orange, peeled, cut into round slices
- ¾ tablespoon coconut oil
- 2 cups chopped collard greens
- ½ teaspoon turmeric powder
- 1 green onion, use only greens, sliced
- 1 tablespoon unsweetened coconut flakes, toasted
- ⅛ cup red lentils, rinsed well, soaked in water for an hour, drained, dried with paper towels

NUTRITIONAL VALUES
PER SERVING:

Calories	314
Fat	17 g
Carbohydrates	35 g
Protein	10 g
Sodium	314 mg
Potassium	589 mg
Phosphorus	125 mg

DIRECTIONS:

1. Make sure the lentils are really dry.
2. Pour sunflower oil into a nonstick skillet and let it heat over medium-high heat. Once oil melts, swirl the pan to spread the oil. Scatter lentils in the pan and cook for a few minutes until they turn crisp. Remove the lentils onto a plate. Sprinkle pepper and toss well.
3. Add coconut oil into the skillet. Once oil melts, add jalapeño and cook for about a minute.
4. Stir in mustard, collard greens, salt, and turmeric and cook for a couple of minutes until the greens wilt a bit. Turn off the heat. Add lentils and stir.
5. Stir in the mint, orange, green onion, and lime juice lightly.
6. Serve garnished with coconut.

159. ZUCCHINI RIBBON PITA PIZZA

Prep. time: 10 min | Cooking time: 10 min | Servings: 2

INGREDIENTS:

- 1 zucchini (about 7 ounces), peeled into ribbons using a vegetable peeler
- ½ teaspoon dried oregano
- 2 pita breads (6 ounces each)
- ½ cup shredded part-skim, low sodium mozzarella cheese
- ⅛ cup thinly sliced ribbons
- ½ tablespoon olive oil
- ⅛ teaspoon freshly ground black pepper
- 3 tablespoons low-sodium tomato sauce
- 1 tablespoon crumbled feta cheese
- 1 tablespoon pine nuts (optional)

NUTRITIONAL VALUES PER SERVING: 2 SPRING ROLLS (WITHOUT DRESSING OR DIP)	
Calories	340
Fat	15 g
Carbohydrates	38 g
Protein	14 g
Sodium	399 mg
Potassium	257 mg
Phosphorus	358 mg

DIRECTIONS:

1. Preheat the oven to 425°F.
2. Place zucchini ribbons in a bowl. Drizzle oil over it. Sprinkle pepper and oregano and toss well.
3. Smear 2 tablespoons of tomato sauce on each pita and place on a baking sheet. Scatter ¼ cup cheese over each pita.
4. Place half the zucchini ribbons on each pita and place the baking sheet in the oven and bake for 10 minutes. Serve hot.

160. PASTA PRIMAVERA

Prep. time: 5 min | Cooking time: 30-35 min | Servings: 3

INGREDIENTS:

- 6 ounces uncooked pasta
- 7 ounces low-sodium chicken broth
- 2 tablespoons half and half creamer
- ⅛ cup grated parmesan cheese
- 6 ounces frozen mixed vegetables
- 1 tablespoon all-purpose white flour
- ⅛ teaspoon garlic powder

NUTRITIONAL VALUES PER SERVING: 1¾ CUP	
Calories	216
Fat	14 g
Carbohydrates	16 g
Protein	7 g
Sodium	318 mg
Potassium	232 mg
Phosphorus	123 mg

DIRECTIONS:

1. Cook the pasta following the directions on the package but do not add salt while cooking.
2. Cook the vegetables following the directions on the package.
3. Combine broth and flour in a pot and place the pot over medium-low heat. Keep whisking until smooth.
4. Whisk in garlic powder and half and half. Whisk well.
5. Cook on low heat until slightly thick. Stir every 2-3 minutes.
6. Stir in pasta and vegetables. Heat thoroughly.
7. Divide pasta into 3 plates. Garnish with parmesan cheese and serve.

161. GRILLED SUMMER VEGETABLES WITH POLENTA

Prep. time: 15 min | Cooking time: 50-60 min | Servings: 2

INGREDIENTS:

- 6 tablespoons milk
- 1 clove garlic, minced
- A pinch sea salt
- 3 sage leaves, divided
- ½ medium zucchini, halved lengthwise, sliced crosswise into 1 inch pieces
- 1 medium shallot, halved
- Freshly ground pepper to taste
- 1 cup water
- ⅓ cup polenta
- 1 tablespoon unsalted butter
- 1 small carrot, peeled, halved lengthwise
- 1 mini bell pepper, halved, deseeded
- 1 tablespoon olive oil
- Greens of 1 small scallion, thinly sliced

NUTRITIONAL VALUES PER SERVING: 1¼ CUPS

Calories	210
Fat	15 g
Carbohydrates	18 g
Protein	4 g
Sodium	182 mg
Potassium	398 mg
Phosphorus	96 mg

DIRECTIONS:

1. Pour milk and water into a saucepan. Add garlic and place the saucepan over high heat.
2. When it starts boiling, add salt and polenta in a thin stream, whisking constantly while adding.
3. Lower the heat and cover the saucepan. Cook for about 7-8 minutes. Do not stir during this time.
4. Uncover and whisk well. If there are any lumps, break them by whisking. Cover the saucepan once again and cook for 10-15 minutes.
5. Add butter into a skillet and place the skillet over medium heat. When butter melts, place one sage leaf and shake the pan often until you can see milk solids separated in the butter. Slowly, the butter will become light brown. Turn off the heat. Remove the sage and keep the butter aside in a bowl. Discard the sage leaf.
6. Place all the vegetables in a bowl. Drizzle oil over the veggies and toss well. Sprinkle pepper and mix well.
7. You can grill the vegetables on a grill pan or on a grill. Preheat a grill to medium-high heat, if you are using the grill and grill for 5-7 minutes on each side. If you are grilling in a grill pan, grill for 5-7 minutes on each side.
8. Remove the grilled vegetables and place on a plate. Let it sit for 3-4 minutes.
9. Meanwhile, divide the polenta equally into 2 bowls. Place the vegetables over the polenta. Place a sage leaf on top in each bowl. Drizzle brown butter over the vegetables and serve garnished with scallions.

162. CREAMY KOHLRABI WITH QUINOA

Prep. time: 10 min | Cooking time: 35-40 min | Servings: 3

INGREDIENTS:

- ⅓ cup quinoa, rinsed
- 1 tablespoon unsalted butter
- ¼ cup water
- ½ teaspoon ground nutmeg
- Freshly ground pepper to taste
- ¼ cup chopped pecans, toasted
- 1 small kohlrabi with leaves
- (green or purple), cut into 1 inch cubes, chop the leaves as well
- ½ medium onion, thinly sliced
- 1 tablespoon minced sage
- ¼ cup heavy cream
- ⅛ teaspoon sea salt
- 1 teaspoon truffle oil (optional)

NUTRITIONAL VALUES PER SERVING: ¾ CUP
(WITHOUT TRUFFLE OIL)

Calories	236
Fat	16 g
Carbohydrates	21 g
Protein	5 g
Sodium	121 mg
Potassium	462 mg
Phosphorus	155 mg

DIRECTIONS:

1. Cook quinoa following the instructions on the package. Keep it aside.
2. Place a pan over medium-high heat. Add butter and allow it to melt. When butter melts, add kohlrabi cubes and onion and stir. Lower the heat to medium-low heat and cook until brown.
3. Pour ¼ cup water and cover the pan. Simmer until kohlrabi is cooked through.
4. Now stir the kohlrabi greens into the pan and cook until they wilt.
5. Add sage, heavy cream, nutmeg, salt, and pepper and mix well. Let it simmer for a couple of minutes. Add some water if you find the sauce very thick. Turn off the heat.
6. Stir in pecans and truffle oil.
7. Divide quinoa into 3 bowls. Divide the kohlrabi mixture among the bowls and serve.

163. COTTAGE CHEESE PANCAKES WITH FRESH STRAWBERRIES

Prep. time: 10 min | Cooking time: 3-4 min per pancake | Servings: 3

INGREDIENTS:

- ½ cup cottage cheese
- ¼ cup all-purpose flour
- 1 ½ cups sliced strawberries
- 2 eggs, lightly beaten
- 3 tablespoons unsalted butter, melted

NUTRITIONAL VALUES PER SERVING: 2 PANCAKES WITH ½ CUP STRAWBERRIES

Calories	216
Fat	14 g
Carbohydrates	16 g
Protein	7 g
Sodium	318 mg
Potassium	232 mg
Phosphorus	123 mg

DIRECTIONS:

1. Place cottage cheese, beaten egg, butter, and flour in a bowl and whisk well.
2. Place a griddle or pan over medium heat. Spray with cooking spray.
3. Pour ¼ cup of batter on the pan. Cook until the underside is browned as per your desire. Turn the pancakes over and cook the other side as well.
4. Remove the pancake from the pan and keep warm.
5. Make the remaining pancakes similarly.
6. Scatter ¼ cup strawberries on each pancake and serve.

164. RICE SALAD

Prep. time: 20 min | Cooking time: 10-12 min | Servings: 6

INGREDIENTS:

DRESSING:
- 4 teaspoons miso paste
- 2 tablespoons olive oil
- 2 cloves garlic, minced
- 2 teaspoons apple cider vinegar
- 4 teaspoons maple syrup
- Juice of 4 limes
- 1 jalapeño, deseeded, chopped

SALAD:
- 8 ounces brown basmati rice
- 4 large carrots, grated
- 2 tablespoons sesame seeds
- ¼ cup chopped cilantro
- 1 medium yellow squash, quartered lengthwise, cut into slices crosswise
- 4 green onions, sliced
- ¼ cup torn mint leaves

NUTRITIONAL VALUES PER SERVING: 2 CUPS	
Calories	258
Fat	8 g
Carbohydrates	44 g
Protein	5 g
Sodium	150 mg
Potassium	496 mg
Phosphorus	188 mg

DIRECTIONS:

1. To make dressing: Place all the dressing ingredients in a blender. Blend the mixture for about 30-40 seconds until you get smooth dressing.
2. Follow the directions on the package and cook brown rice.
3. Pour enough water into a pot such that it is about 2 inches in height from the bottom of the pot. Place the pot over high heat and let it start boiling.
4. Place squash in a steamer basket and place the basket in the pot. Cover the steamer basket and cook for 4 minutes or until cooked through.
5. Place rice, squash, green onions, carrots, and sesame seeds in a large bowl and toss well.
6. Add dressing and mix well.
7. Serve in bowls garnished with mint and cilantro leaves.

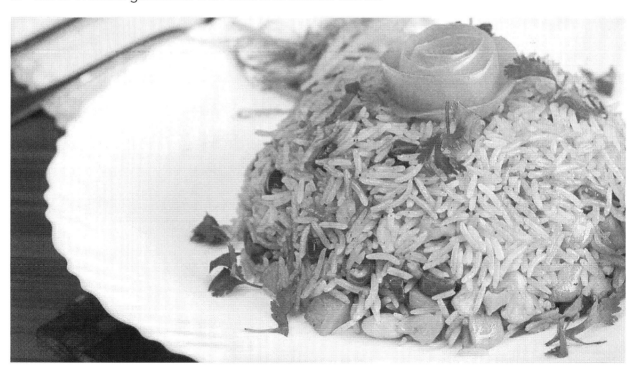

165. CHAYOTE VEGAN CEVICHE

Prep. time: 15 min | Cooking time: 15 min + chilling time | Servings: 3

INGREDIENTS:

- 1 medium chayote squash
- ⅛ cup orange juice
- ½ cup lime juice
- 1 tablespoon olive oil
- ½ teaspoon cayenne pepper
- ½ cup chopped tomatoes
- ½ jalapeño pepper, chopped
- ¼ cup corn kernels
- ⅛ teaspoon sea salt
- ½ avocado, peeled, pitted, diced
- ½ medium red onion, chopped
- 2 medium radish, chopped
- ½ cup chopped ripe mango
- ¼ cup chopped cilantro

NUTRITIONAL VALUES PER SERVING: 1 CUP (WITHOUT TORTILLA CHIPS)	
Calories	162
Fat	9 g
Carbohydrates	23 g
Protein	2 g
Sodium	109 mg
Potassium	536 mg
Phosphorus	73 mg

DIRECTIONS:

1. Boil chayote in a pot of water for about 15-20 minutes or until fork tender.
2. Drain the water and immerse in a bowl of ice water. Now peel the skin and remove the seeds. Cut into ½ inch cubes.
3. To make marinade: Combine orange juice, lime juice, oil, cayenne pepper, and salt in a bowl and whisk well.
4. Add chayote, cilantro, vegetables, and fruits and toss well. Cover the bowl and chill for 30-60 minutes.
5. Serve with low-sodium corn or flour tortilla chips.

166. MEDITERRANEAN GREEN BEANS

Prep. time: 10 min | Cooking time: 10 min per pancake | Servings: 2

INGREDIENTS:

- ½ pound fresh green beans, stringed, cut into 1 ½ inch pieces
- 1 ¼ teaspoons olive oil
- ⅔ cup water
- 1 ½ tablespoons fresh lemon juice
- 2 cloves garlic, peeled, minced
- A pinch pepper

NUTRITIONAL VALUES PER SERVING: 1 CUP	
Calories	71
Fat	3 g
Carbohydrates	10 g
Protein	2 g
Sodium	2 mg
Potassium	186 mg
Phosphorus	37 mg

DIRECTIONS:

1. Pour water into a skillet and bring it to boil over medium-high heat. When it begins to boil, add beans and let it boil for 3 minutes. Drain in a colander.
2. Place the skillet back over heat. Once the pan is dry, pour oil. When the oil is hot, add beans and garlic and cook for a minute. Stir in the juice and pepper stir-fry for a minute.
3. Serve hot.

167. VEGETABLE CASSEROLE

Prep. time: 5 min | Cooking time: 3-4 min | Servings: 1

INGREDIENTS:

- ½ teaspoon olive oil
- ¼ cup canned low-sodium green beans
- A pinch pepper
- A pinch paprika
- ¼ cup cubed yellow summer squash
- 4 ounces All whites liquid whites

NUTRITIONAL VALUES PER SERVING	
Calories	76
Fat	0 g
Carbohydrates	5 g
Protein	14 g
Sodium	207 mg
Potassium	344 mg
Phosphorus	344 mg

DIRECTIONS:

1. Grease a small microwave safe container with ½ teaspoon oil.
2. Spread the squash and green beans in the dish.
3. Drizzle All Whites liquid whites over the vegetables. Add pepper and paprika.
4. Cover the dish and place in a microwave. Cook on High for 3-4 minutes or until the liquid whites are cooked. Stir once halfway through cooking.
5. To cook in a pan: Cook squash in oil, in a pan until slightly tender.
6. Add beans and cook for a few minutes until squash is tender.
7. Add All Whites liquid egg white, pepper, and paprika and stir. Cook covered for 5-8 minutes until set in the center.

168. ITALIAN EGGPLANT SALAD

Prep. time: 10 min | Cooking time: 20 min | Servings: 2

INGREDIENTS:

- 1 ½ cups cubed eggplant
- 1 tablespoon white wine vinegar
- ¼ teaspoon oregano
- 1 small tomato, chopped
- ½ small onion, chopped
- 2 small cloves garlic, chopped
- ⅛ teaspoon pepper
- 1 ½ tablespoons olive oil

NUTRITIONAL VALUES PER SERVING: ½ CUP	
Calories	69
Fat	5 g
Carbohydrates	6 g
Protein	1 g
Sodium	2 mg
Potassium	118 mg
Phosphorus	15 mg

DIRECTIONS:

1. Boil water in a pot over high heat. Add eggplant. When it begins to boil again, lower the heat and cook until tender.
2. Drain in a colander and place in a glass dish.
3. Add onion and stir.
4. Add vinegar, pepper, and garlic into a bowl and whisk well. Drizzle over the eggplant mixture. Stir well.
5. Add oil just before serving. Stir and serve.

169. CAULIFLOWER WITH WHOLE-WHEAT BREADCRUMBS

Prep. time: 5 min I Cooking time: 20 min I Servings: 2

INGREDIENTS:

- ½ slice whole-wheat bread
- ⅛ teaspoon salt
- A pinch black pepper
- ½ medium head cauliflower, cut into florets
- ½ tablespoon soft tub margarine

NUTRITIONAL VALUES PER SERVING: 1 CUP	
Calories	45
Fat	4 g
Carbohydrates	5 g
Protein	2 g
Sodium	120 mg
Potassium	152 mg
Phosphorus	171 mg

DIRECTIONS:

1. Toast the bread piece in a toaster at the lowest setting. Each time it pops up, toast it again until crisp and not burnt.
2. Pour enough water into a pot such that it is about 2 inches in height from the bottom of the pot. Place the pot over high heat and let it start boiling.
3. Place cauliflower florets in a steamer basket and place the basket in the pot. Cover the steamer basket and cook for 5-8 minutes or until fork tender, making sure not to overcook.
4. Tear up the toasted bread and place in a blender. Give short pulses until medium size crumbs are formed.
5. Add margarine into a pan and place the pan over medium heat. When margarine melts, stir breadcrumbs into the margarine. Add pepper and cook for a few minutes until light-medium brown in color. Add cauliflower and salt and mix well. Heat thoroughly.
6. Serve hot.

170. MOROCCAN COUSCOUS

NUTRITIONAL VALUES PER SERVING: ½ CUP	
Calories	126
Fat	2 g
Carbohydrates	23 g
Protein	4 g
Sodium	5.5 mg
Potassium	57 mg
Phosphorus	51 mg

Prep. time: 3 min I Cooking time: 10 min I Servings: 2

INGREDIENTS:

- 1 tablespoon chopped onion
- ½ cup water
- ⅓ cup dry couscous
- ¾ teaspoon olive oil

DIRECTIONS:

1. Add oil into a pan and heat it over medium heat. When oil is hot, add onion and cook until soft. Turn off the heat.
2. Pour water into a saucepan and place the saucepan over high heat. When it starts boiling, turn off the heat.
3. Add onion and couscous and stir. Cover the saucepan and let it rest for 5 minutes.
4. Take a fork and fluff the couscous.
5. Serve.

171. SPRING ONION FLATBREAD

Prep. time: 1 hour and 30 min | Cooking time: 6 min per flatbread | Servings: 2

INGREDIENTS:

- 1 ½ cups unbleached flour
- A tiny pinch sea salt
- 2-3 spring onions, chopped
- 1 teaspoon dried yeast
- ¾ cup water
- 1 tablespoon sunflower oil

NUTRITIONAL VALUES PER SERVING: 1 FLATBREAD	
Calories	413
Fat	8 g
Carbohydrates	74 g
Protein	11 g
Sodium	78 mg
Potassium	169 mg
Phosphorus	120 mg

DIRECTIONS:

1. Combine flour, salt, and yeast in a mixing bowl. Make a big cavity in the center of the flour mixture and add water into it.
2. Mix well into a dough using your hands.
3. Dust your countertop with some flour. Place the dough on your countertop and knead for a couple of minutes. Cover the dough and let it rest for 15 minutes.
4. Knead the dough once again for 5 minutes.
5. Place the dough in a greased bowl. Turn the dough around in the bowl to grease the dough and cover the bowl. Place the bowl in a warm area for 30 minutes.
6. Grease your countertop lightly with some cooking spray. Place the dough on the greased area and flatten the dough with your hand.
7. Scatter spring onions over the dough. Fold the dough over the spring onions and make sure to knead the dough for another 3 minutes.
8. Make 2 equal portions of the dough and shape into balls. Cover the dough and keep it aside for 30 minutes.
9. Now grease your hands with some oil. Take a ball of dough and form into a disc of about 10 inches diameter that is thin in the center and thick around the edges, by pulling and stretching the dough.
10. Place a large pan or griddle over medium-high heat. Brush oil on the pan.
11. Place the flatbread on the griddle. Let it cook for a couple of minutes. Brush oil on top of the flatbread as well. Lift the underside and check if it is cooked, you should have a few brown spots. Turn the flatbread over and cook the other side until it has a few spots on it.
12. Remove from the pan and serve.
13. Make the other flatbread similarly (steps 9-11).

172. SAUTÉED COLLARD GREENS

Prep. time: 10 min | Cooking time: 15 min | Servings: 3

INGREDIENTS:

- 4 cups chopped, fresh collard greens
- ½ tablespoon unsalted butter
- ½ tablespoon chopped garlic
- ½ teaspoon pepper
- 1 tablespoon olive oil
- 2 tablespoons minced onions
- ½ teaspoon crushed red pepper flakes
- ½ tablespoon vinegar (optional)

NUTRITIONAL VALUES PER SERVING: ⅓ OF THE RECIPE	
Calories	79
Fat	5 g
Carbohydrates	4 g
Protein	2 g
Sodium	9 mg
Potassium	129 mg
Phosphorus	18 mg

DIRECTIONS:

1. Place a pot of water over high heat. When it begins to boil, add collard greens and blanch for 30 seconds.
2. Drain and place in a bowl of chilled water. Drain off after 5-6 minutes.
3. Add butter and oil into a skillet and place it over medium-high heat. When the butter melts, add garlic and onions and sauté until light brown.
4. Raise high heat. Stir the collard greens, red pepper flakes, and pepper into the onion mixture and cook for 4-5 minutes. Turn off the heat.
5. Add vinegar if using and toss well.
6. Serve hot.

173. KOHLRABI SALAD WITH CILANTRO DRESSING

Prep. time: 15 min | Cooking time: 0 min | Servings: 2

INGREDIENTS:

- ½ medium kohlrabi, trimmed, peeled, thinly sliced
- 1.8 ounce sweet mini peppers, cut into ¼ inch thick slices
- 2 medium Bibb lettuce leaves
- ½ small pear, peeled, cored
- ½ jalapeño pepper, sliced

SALAD:
- ⅛ cup chopped cilantro
- Juice of a lime
- ¼ teaspoon honey
- A tiny pinch sea salt
- 1 ¼ tablespoons olive oil
- ½ small clove garlic, minced
- ⅛ teaspoon ground cumin

NUTRITIONAL VALUES PER SERVING: ¾ CUP	
Calories	134
Fat	9 g
Carbohydrates	14 g
Protein	2 g
Sodium	56 mg
Potassium	409 mg
Phosphorus	51 mg

DIRECTIONS:

1. Make a pile of the kohlrabi slices and cut into ½ inch wide strips.
2. Similarly, make a pile of pear slices and cut into ½ inch wide strips.
3. Combine kohlrabi, pear, jalapeño, and peppers in a bowl.
4. Combine all the dressing ingredients in a bowl and pour over the salad. Toss well.
5. Divide the salad among the lettuce leaves and serve.

174. ENDIVE, PEAR AND GORGONZOLA SALAD

Prep. time: 10 min | Cooking time: 0 min | Servings: 2

INGREDIENTS:

- ½ teaspoon olive oil
- ¼ cup canned low-sodium green beans
- A pinch pepper
- ¼ cup cubed yellow summer
- squash
- 4 ounces All whites liquid whites
- A pinch paprika

NUTRITIONAL VALUES PER SERVING: ½ THE RECIPE	
Calories	76
Fat	0 g
Carbohydrates	5 g
Protein	14 g
Sodium	207 mg
Potassium	344 mg
Phosphorus	344 mg

DIRECTIONS:

1. Grease a small microwave safe container with ½ teaspoon oil.
2. Spread the squash and green beans in the dish.
3. Drizzle All Whites liquid whites over the vegetables. Add pepper and paprika.
4. Cover the dish and place in a microwave. Cook on High for 3-4 minutes or until the liquid whites are cooked. Stir once halfway through cooking.
5. To cook in a pan: Cook squash in oil, in a pan until slightly tender.
6. Add beans and cook for a few minutes until squash is tender.
7. Add All Whites liquid egg white, pepper, and paprika and stir. Cook covered for 5-8 minutes until set in the center.

175. BBQ ASPARAGUS

Prep. time: 10 min | Cooking time: 5 min | Servings: 3

INGREDIENTS:

- ¾ pound fresh asparagus, trimmed
- ¾ teaspoon pepper
- 1 ½ tablespoons extra-virgin olive oil
- 1 ½ tablespoons lemon juice

NUTRITIONAL VALUES PER SERVING: ⅓ RECIPE	
Calories	86
Fat	6 g
Carbohydrates	5 g
Protein	3 g
Sodium	4 mg
Potassium	196 mg
Phosphorus	41 mg

DIRECTIONS:

1. Add oil, lemon juice, and pepper into a shallow, wide dish. Place the asparagus in the bowl. Roll the asparagus around so that the asparagus is well coated with the mixture.
2. Chill until you prepare the grill.
3. Preheat a grill to medium-high heat. Spray some cooking spray inside the grill basket or line with aluminum foil and grease a vegetable grilling tray.
4. Place the asparagus in the grill tray or basket and grill until light brown. Stir often.
5. Remove onto a plate. Cool for a couple of minutes and serve.

176. WATERMELON FETA SALAD

Prep. time: 10 min | Cooking time: 0 min | Servings: 2

INGREDIENTS:

- 2 cups watermelon cubes (½ inch cubes)
- 1 tablespoon chopped mint
- 1 tablespoon olive oil
- 1 teaspoon honey
- 3 tablespoons crumbled feta cheese
- ½ teaspoon minced onion
- 1 tablespoon red wine vinegar

NUTRITIONAL VALUES PER SERVING: ABOUT 1 CUP	
Calories	152
Fat	10 g
Carbohydrates	15 g
Protein	3 g
Sodium	144 mg
Potassium	197 mg
Phosphorus	61 mg

DIRECTIONS:

1. Whisk together oil, honey, and vinegar in a small bowl.
2. Add watermelon, onion, mint, and feta cheese into a bowl and toss well.
3. Pour dressing over the salad. Toss well and serve.

177. GARLIC MASHED POTATOES

Prep. time: 5 min | Cooking time: 20 min | Servings: 2

INGREDIENTS:

- 1 medium potato, peeled, cut into small pieces
- 2 tablespoons butter
- 1-2 cloves garlic, peeled, sliced
- ⅛ cup 1% low-fat milk

NUTRITIONAL VALUES PER SERVING: ½ CUP	
Calories	185
Fat	13 g
Carbohydrates	15 g
Protein	2 g
Sodium	103 mg
Potassium	205 mg
Phosphorus	65 mg

DIRECTIONS:

1. Drop potato and garlic into a pot of boiling water over medium heat, until soft. Drain in a colander. Place in a bowl.
2. Beat the potato mixture with an electric hand mixer until creamy.
3. Add butter and milk and beat until smooth.
4. If you want to reduce the potassium in the potatoes, double boil the potatoes. For this, cut the potatoes into small pieces. Pour water into a saucepan. Add garlic and potatoes and place the saucepan over medium heat.
5. When water starts boiling, discard the boiling water and pour more water into the pot. Cook until soft.

178. RICE AND VERMICELLI PILAF

Prep. time: 5 min | Cooking time: 20-25 min | Servings: 2-3

INGREDIENTS:

- 1 ounce vermicelli noodles, break into 1 inch pieces
- ½ cup uncooked parboiled rice
- ½ tablespoon Mrs. Dash onion and herb seasoning
- blend
- 1 tablespoon unsalted butter
- 1 cup water
- ½ teaspoon chicken bouillon granules

NUTRITIONAL VALUES PER SERVING: ¾ CUP	
Calories	188
Fat	4 g
Carbohydrates	34 g
Protein	4 g
Sodium	137 mg
Potassium	118 mg
Phosphorus	80 mg

DIRECTIONS:

1. Add ½ tablespoon butter into a skillet and melt it over medium heat. When butter melts, add vermicelli and stir-fry until light brown.
2. Add ½ tablespoon butter and rice and mix well. Cook for a couple of minutes.
3. Stir in seasoning and bouillon granules. Pour water and mix well.
4. Cook covered over medium heat until tender. Remove from heat and let it rest for 5 minutes.
5. Uncover the pan and loosen the pilaf with a fork.
6. Serve hot.

179. SEASONED CABBAGE STEAKS

Prep. time: 5 min | Cooking time: 60 min | Servings: 3

INGREDIENTS:

- ½ medium head cabbage (make sure to cut a whole medium cabbage lengthwise, from stem side downwards, into 2 halves and use one half)
- ¼ teaspoon pepper
- ½ tablespoon minced fresh dill
- ½ tablespoon salt-free seasoning of your choice
- 1 tablespoon olive oil

NUTRITIONAL VALUES PER SERVING: ⅓ RECIPE	
Calories	90
Fat	5 g
Carbohydrates	9 g
Protein	2 g
Sodium	26 mg
Potassium	267 mg
Phosphorus	38 mg

DIRECTIONS:

1. Hold the cabbage on your cutting board and cut into 3 thick slices of 1 inch each. Start from the stem side and go down straight to the other end while cutting. These are your cabbage steaks.
2. Brush oil over the cabbage steaks and place on a greased baking sheet.
3. Sprinkle dill, pepper, and seasoning over the cabbage and keep the baking sheet covered with aluminum foil.
4. Preheat the oven to 350°F. Place the baking sheet in the oven and set the timer for 45 minutes.
5. Uncover and continue baking for 15 minutes or until brown at a few spots.

180. CABBAGE, ONION, AND SWEET PEPPER MEDLEY

Prep. time: 10 min | Cooking time: 10-12 min | Servings: 2

INGREDIENTS:

• 2 cups watermelon cubes (½ inch cubes)	• 3 tablespoons crumbled feta cheese
• 1 tablespoon chopped mint	• ½ teaspoon minced onion
• 1 tablespoon olive oil	• 1 tablespoon red wine vinegar
• 1 teaspoon honey	

NUTRITIONAL VALUES PER SERVING: ½ THE RECIPE

Calories	70
Fat	4 g
Carbohydrates	8 g
Protein	1 g
Sodium	52 mg
Potassium	208 mg
Phosphorus	29 mg

DIRECTIONS:

1. Add onion, cabbage, and bell peppers into a nonstick pan and place the pan over high heat. Stir-fry for a couple of minutes.
2. Whisk together vinegar, oil, mustard, pepper, and brown sugar in a bowl and pour it into the pan. Mix well. Cook for a few minutes until the vegetables are crisp as well as tender.
3. Divide into 2 equal portions and serve.

181. SWEET AND CRUNCHY COLESLAW

Prep. time: 10 min | Cooking time: 0 min + chilling time | Servings: 6

INGREDIENTS:

• 3 cups shredded cabbage	• ½ cup sugar
• ½ teaspoons celery seeds	• ¼ cup chopped sweet onion
• ½ teaspoon prepared yellow mustard	• ½ cup canola oil
	• ¼ cup rice vinegar

NUTRITIONAL VALUES PER SERVING: ½ CUP

Calories	244
Fat	19 g
Carbohydrates	20 g
Protein	1 g
Sodium	12 mg
Potassium	73 mg
Phosphorus	13 mg

DIRECTIONS:

1. Combine onion and cabbage in a bowl.
2. Place sugar, celery seeds, mustard, oil, and vinegar in a blender and blend until sugar dissolves completely and the mixture is smooth.
3. Pour the blended mixture over the vegetables and toss well.
4. Chill until use.

182. KALE SLAW

Prep. time: 15 min | Cooking time: 15 min + chilling time | Servings: 3

INGREDIENTS:

- ¼ bunch fresh kale, discard hard ribs and stems, finely chopped
- 3 medium Brussels sprouts, shredded
- 1 tablespoon shallots
- 3 tablespoons dried, sweetened cranberries
- 1 ½ tablespoons cider vinegar
- ½ teaspoon Mrs. Dash garlic and herb seasoning
- A pinch pepper
- 1 ½ tablespoons olive oil
- 1 ½ tablespoons honey
- ¼ teaspoon yellow mustard

NUTRITIONAL VALUES
PER SERVING: ½ CUP

Calories	143
Fat	7 g
Carbohydrates	18 g
Protein	2 g
Sodium	29 mg
Potassium	245 mg
Phosphorus	38 mg

DIRECTIONS:

1. Place kale, cranberries, brussels sprouts, and shallots in a bowl and toss well.
2. Whisk together the rest of the ingredients in a bowl.
3. Pour over the vegetables. Toss well. Chill for 30 minutes and serve.

183. MASHED CARROTS AND GINGER

Prep. time: 10 min | Cooking time: 15 min | Servings: 6

INGREDIENTS:

- 4 cups baby carrots
- 1 teaspoon honey
- 1 teaspoon vanilla extract
- 1 teaspoon minced ginger
- 1 teaspoon pepper
- 2 tablespoons chopped chives (optional)

NUTRITIONAL VALUES
PER SERVING: ⅙ RECIPE

Calories	30
Fat	0 g
Carbohydrates	7 g
Protein	1 g
Sodium	55 mg
Potassium	174 mg
Phosphorus	21 mg

DIRECTIONS:

1. Pour enough water into a pot such that it is about 2 inches in height from the bottom of the pot. Place the pot over high heat and let it start boiling.
2. Place carrots in a steamer basket and place the basket in the pot. Cover the steamer basket and cook for 10 minutes or until soft.
3. Transfer the carrots into a bowl and mash them using a potato masher until the texture you desire is achieved. If you want a smooth texture, you can blend with an immersion blender.
4. Stir in honey, vanilla, ginger, pepper, and chives if using and stir.

CHAPTER 10

Snack Recipes

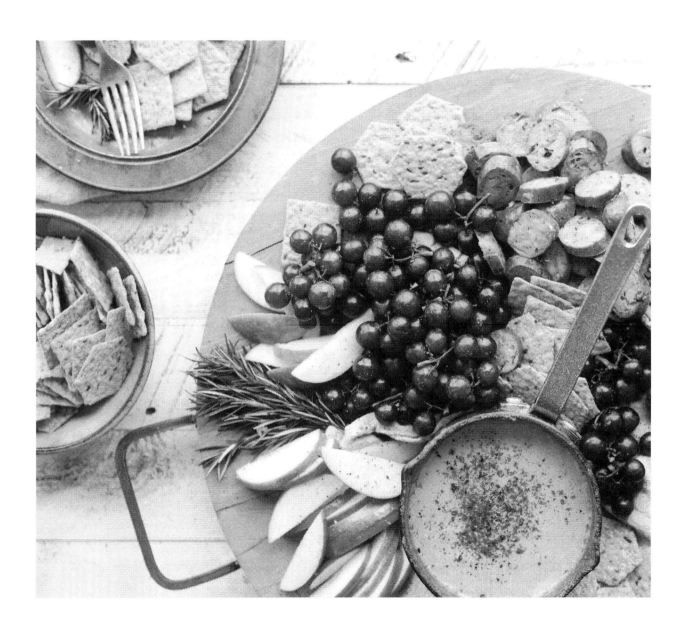

184. WATERMELON AND CUCUMBER SMOOTHIE

Prep. time: 10 min | Cooking time: 0 min | Servings: 2

INGREDIENTS:

NUTRITIONAL VALUES PER SERVING: 1 GLASS	
Calories	54
Fat	0 g
Carbohydrates	13 g
Protein	1 g
Sodium	7 mg
Potassium	263 mg
Phosphorus	52 mg

- 2 cups chopped, deseeded watermelon
- Ice cubes, as required
- 4 teaspoons agave nectar (optional)
- 1 cup peeled, chopped cucumber
- Juice of a lime
- Few mint leaves, to garnish

DIRECTIONS:

1. Add watermelon, ice cubes, agave nectar, cucumber, and lime juice into a high-speed blender.
2. Blend for 35-50 seconds or until smooth.
3. Pour into 2 glasses and serve.

185. BLUEBERRY AND PINAPPLE SMOOTHIE

Prep. time: 5 min | Cooking time: 0 min | Servings: 1

INGREDIENTS:

NUTRITIONAL VALUES PER SERVING: ½ CUP	
Calories	155.4
Fat	0.75 g
Carbohydrates	31.1 g
Protein	7.4 g
Sodium	104.1 mg
Potassium	289.4 mg
Phosphorus	289.4 mg

- ⅓ cup + 1 tablespoon pineapple juice
- 4 tablespoons pasteurized egg whites
- ⅔ teaspoon sugar or splenda
- 2-3 tablespoons water or more if required
- ⅔ cup frozen blueberries, slightly defrosted

DIRECTIONS:

1. Add pineapple juice, egg whites, water, blueberries, and sweetener into a high speed blender.
2. Blend for 35-50 seconds or until smooth. Pour into a tall glass. Serve with crushed ice if desired.

186. STRAWBERRY APPLE JUICE BLEND

Prep. time: 5 min | Cooking time: 0 min | Servings: 1

INGREDIENTS:

NUTRITIONAL VALUES PER SERVING: 6 OUNCES	
Calories	84
Fat	0 g
Carbohydrates	20 g
Protein	1 g
Sodium	2 mg
Potassium	238 mg
Phosphorus	30 mg

- ½ cup strawberries
- 3 mint leaves
- 2 ounces green tea
- ½ medium apple
- 1 teaspoon lemon juice

DIRECTIONS:

1. Juice together apple, strawberries, and mint leaves in a juicer.
2. Pour juice into a cup. Add lemon juice and green tea and stir.
3. Serve at room temperature or add ice and serve chilled.

187. HAZELNUT CINNAMON COFFEE

Prep. time: 2 min | Cooking time: 2 min | Servings: 2

INGREDIENTS:

- 2 cups brewed coffee
- 2 tablespoons 1% low-fat milk
- 4 teaspoons Torani Sugar-free Classic Hazelnut Syrup
- 2 sticks cinnamon

NUTRITIONAL VALUES
PER SERVING: 1 CUP

Calories	13
Fat	0 g
Carbohydrates	1 g
Protein	1 g
Sodium	13 mg
Potassium	139 mg
Phosphorus	22 mg

DIRECTIONS:

1. Prepare the coffee in a coffee maker as you normally do.
2. Pour brewed coffee into 2 cups. Pour 2 teaspoons of hazelnut syrup and a tablespoon of milk into each cup and stir. Place a stick of cinnamon on top in each cup and serve.

188. APPLE-CINNAMON FLAVORED WATER

Prep. time: 5 min | Cooking time: 0 min + chilling time | Servings: 5

INGREDIENTS:

- 5 cups water
- 1 stick cinnamon
- 1 teaspoon ground cinnamon
- ½ medium apple, cored, thinly sliced

NUTRITIONAL VALUES
PER SERVING: ⅙ RECIPE

Calories	4
Fat	0 g
Carbohydrates	1 g
Protein	0 g
Sodium	7 mg
Potassium	10 mg
Phosphorus	0 mg

DIRECTIONS:

1. Add water, cinnamon stick, apple, and ground cinnamon into a pitcher and stir.
2. Place the pitcher in the refrigerator for 8-9 hours.
3. Pour the flavored water into cups and serve.

189. BEET AND APPLE JUICE

Prep. time: 10 min | Cooking time: 0 min | Servings: 1

INGREDIENTS:

- ¼ medium apple, sliced
- ½ medium carrot, sliced
- A handful parsley
- ¼ medium beet, sliced
- ½ stalk celery, sliced

NUTRITIONAL VALUES
PER SERVING: 3 OUNCES

Calories	53
Fat	0 g
Carbohydrates	13 g
Protein	1 g
Sodium	66 mg
Potassium	338 mg
Phosphorus	36 mg

DIRECTIONS:

1. Juice together apple, carrot, parsley, beet and celery in a juicer.
2. Pour into a cup and serve.

190. LEMON COOLER

Prep. time: 5 min | Cooking time: 0 min | Servings: 2

INGREDIENTS:

- 8 large ice cubes
- ½ cup half and half creamer
- 2 tablespoons lemon juice
- 6 tablespoons sugar
- 2 thin lemon wedges to garnish

NUTRITIONAL VALUES PER SERVING: 6 OUNCES	
Calories	230
Fat	7 g
Carbohydrates	40 g
Protein	2 g
Sodium	25 mg
Potassium	91 mg
Phosphorus	58 mg

DIRECTIONS:

1. Place ice cubes, half and half creamer, lemon juice, and sugar in a blender.
2. Set the blender on ice or crush option and blend until you get slush.
3. Divide into 2 glasses. Top with a lemon wedge in each glass and serve.

191. STRAWBERRY LEMONADE SLUSH

Prep. time: 5 min | Cooking time: 0 min | Servings: 2

INGREDIENTS:

- ⅔ cup fresh lemon juice
- 2 tablespoons sugar
- 1 cup ice cubes
- 1 cup fresh or frozen strawberries

NUTRITIONAL VALUES PER SERVING: 1 CUP	
Calories	128
Fat	0 g
Carbohydrates	33 g
Protein	0 g
Sodium	2 mg
Potassium	148 mg
Phosphorus	20 mg

DIRECTIONS:

1. Place ice cubes, strawberries, lemon juice, and sugar in a blender.
2. Set the blender on ice or crush option and blend until you get slush.
3. Divide into 2 glasses and serve.

192. HUMMUS AND RED PEPPER CELERY LOGS

Prep. time: 5 min | Cooking time: 0 min | Servings: 2

INGREDIENTS:

- 2 celery ribs (8 inches each)
- 2 tablespoons hummus
- 1 tablespoon diced red bell pepper

NUTRITIONAL VALUES PER SERVING: ½ CUP	
Calories	42
Fat	2 g
Carbohydrates	4 g
Protein	2 g
Sodium	89 mg
Potassium	144 mg
Phosphorus	37 mg

DIRECTIONS:

1. Spoon a tablespoon of hummus into each celery rib.
2. Cut each into about 2 ½ inch long pieces. Scatter red bell pepper pieces on top and serve.

193. STUFFED MUSHROOMS

Prep. time: 10 min | Cooking time: 15 min | Servings: 2

INGREDIENTS:

- 4 white mushrooms
- ½ teaspoon balsamic vinegar
- ½ teaspoon oil
- Freshly ground black pepper to taste

FILLING:
- 3 tablespoons low-sodium cheddar cheese
- 2 teaspoons minced cilantro

- 1 ½ tablespoons minced red onion
- 1 teaspoon minced jalapeño pepper
- ½ teaspoon ground coriander
- 1 ½ tablespoons minced red bell pepper
- A tiny pinch sea salt
- ⅛ teaspoon paprika

NUTRITIONAL VALUES PER SERVING: 2 STUFFED MUSHROOMS	
Calories	68
Fat	5 g
Carbohydrates	3 g
Protein	4 g
Sodium	94 mg
Potassium	163 mg
Phosphorus	86 mg

DIRECTIONS:

1. Preheat the oven to 350°F. Prepare a baking sheet by lining it with parchment paper.
2. Wipe the mushrooms with a moist cloth. Carefully remove the mushroom stems.
3. Whisk together oil, pepper, and vinegar in a bowl. Place mushrooms in the bowl and stir well.
4. To make filling: Place spices, salt, jalapeño, cheese, onion, bell pepper, and cilantro in a bowl. Stir until well combined.
5. Make 4 equal portions of the filling and fill into the mushroom caps. Place them on the baking sheet with the filled side facing up.
6. Place the baking sheet in the oven and set the timer for 12 minutes or until mushrooms are cooked and the filling is thoroughly heated.

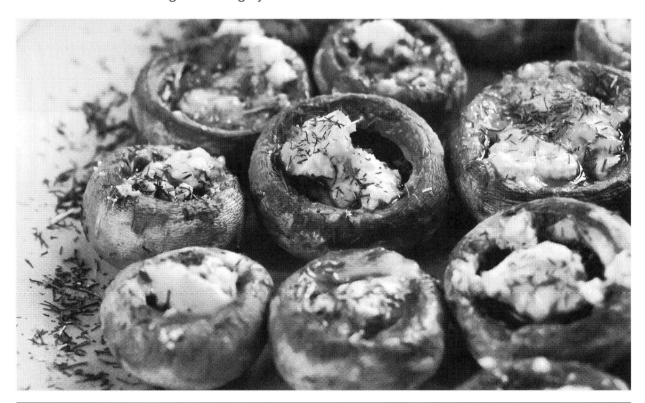

194. TROPICAL SALAD

Prep. time: 15 min | Cooking time: 0 min | Servings: 3

INGREDIENTS:

- 1 ½ cups cubed fresh pineapple
- ½ medium orange bell pepper, diced
- ½ medium jalapeño, diced
- ½ cup arugula
- ½ small red onion, diced
- ½ medium cucumber, halved lengthwise, cut into slices crosswise
- ⅛ cup chopped cilantro

DRESSING:
- 2 tablespoons olive oil
- 1 tablespoon lime juice
- 1 tablespoon honey
- ½ teaspoon cider vinegar
- ⅛ teaspoon freshly ground pepper
- ¼ teaspoon crushed red pepper flakes
- ⅛ teaspoon sea salt

NUTRITIONAL VALUES PER SERVING: 1 CUP	
Calories	160
Fat	9 g
Carbohydrates	21 g
Protein	1 g
Sodium	102 mg
Potassium	230 mg
Phosphorus	26 mg

DIRECTIONS:

Place all the salad ingredients in a bowl and toss well. Whisk together all the dressing ingredients in another bowl and drizzle over the salad. Toss well and serve.

195. SPICY CORNBREAD

Prep. time: 15 min | Cooking time: 30 min | Servings: 16

INGREDIENTS:

- 2 cups all-purpose white flour
- 2 tablespoons sugar
- 2 teaspoons chili powder
- 2 cups plain cornmeal
- 4 teaspoons baking powder
- ½ teaspoon pepper
- 2 cups rice milk, un-enriched
- 2 egg whites
- 2 whole eggs
- 4 tablespoons canola oil
- ½ cup finely grated carrots
- 1 cup finely chopped scallions
- 2 cloves garlic, peeled, minced

NUTRITIONAL VALUES PER SERVING: 1 PIECE (2 x 4 INCHES)	
Calories	188
Fat	5 g
Carbohydrates	31 g
Protein	5 g
Sodium	155 mg
Potassium	100 mg
Phosphorus	81 mg

DIRECTIONS:

1. Preheat the oven to 400°F. Grease a large baking dish (9x13 inches) with cooking spray.
2. Add all the dry ingredients, i.e. flour, sugar, chili powder, cornmeal, baking powder, and pepper into a large mixing bowl and mix until well incorporated.
3. Add rice milk, egg whites, eggs, and oil into the bowl of dry ingredients and mix until just incorporated.
4. Add vegetables and stir. Spoon the batter into the baking dish.
5. Bake the cornbread for about 30 minutes or until the top begins to look golden brown.
6. Remove from the oven and cool for a few minutes.
7. Cut into 16 equal pieces of (2 x 4 inches) and serve.

196. FRIED POTATOES

Prep. time: 30-40 min | Cooking time: 10-12 min | Servings: 2

INGREDIENTS:

- 1 medium potato, peeled, cut into pieces of 4 x ½ inches each (16 pieces in all)
- ¼ teaspoon ground cumin
- A pinch white pepper
- ¼ cup canola oil
- ⅛ teaspoon paprika
- 4 teaspoons low-sodium ketchup

NUTRITIONAL VALUES
PER SERVING: 8 PIECES
(4 x ½ INCHES)

Calories	156
Fat	7 g
Carbohydrates	21 g
Protein	2 g
Sodium	134 mg
Potassium	181 mg
Phosphorus	54 mg

DIRECTIONS:

1. Drop potato pieces into a pot of water and soak for 30 minutes. Drain in a colander. Go to step 4.
2. If you want to reduce the potassium in the potatoes, double boil the potatoes. For this, pour water into a saucepan. Add potatoes and place the saucepan over medium heat.
3. When water starts boiling, discard the boiling water and pour more water into the pot. Cook until fork tender.
4. Pour oil into a skillet and let it heat over medium heat. When oil is hot, add potatoes and cook until golden brown all over.
5. Remove potatoes with a slotted spoon and place on a plate lined with paper towels.
6. Combine all the spices in a small bowl and sprinkle over the potatoes.
7. Divide into 2 plates and serve.

197. WONTON QUICHE MINIS

Prep. time: 35-40 min | Cooking time: 15 min | Servings: 24

INGREDIENTS:

- 2 ounces lean cooked ham, finely chopped
- ¼ cup chopped sweet red bell pepper
- 2 tablespoon all-purpose
- white flour
- ¼ cup chopped green onion
- 10 large eggs
- 48 wonton wrappers (3 ¼ x 3 inches each)

NUTRITIONAL VALUES
PER SERVING: 2 WONTON
QUICHE MINIS

Calories	70
Fat	4 g
Carbohydrates	8 g
Protein	4 g
Sodium	95 mg
Potassium	47 mg
Phosphorus	55 mg

DIRECTIONS:

1. Preheat the oven to 350°F. Grease 48 mini muffin cups with cooking spray. You can use 2-3 mini muffin pans instead of mini muffin cups.
2. Add eggs into a bowl and whisk well. Add ham, bell pepper, flour, and green onion and whisk well.
3. Line each of the muffin cups with a wonton wrapper. Place it such that it lines the bottom as well as the sides of the cup.
4. Divide the egg mixture equally among the muffin cups.
5. Place the muffin cups in the oven and set the timer for about 12-15 minutes. If the muffins are ready, a toothpick when inserted in the middle of muffins should come out clean without any particles stuck on it.
6. Let it cool for a few minutes in the pan. Remove along with the wrappers and serve.

198. CRISPY EGGPLANT FRENCH FRIES

Prep. time: 10 min | Cooking time: 10 min | Servings: 3

INGREDIENTS:

- ½ medium eggplant, peeled, cut into fries (4 x ¾ inches each)
- 1 large egg
- ½ cup 1% low-fat milk
- ¼ cup canola oil
- 6 tablespoons cornstarch
- 6 tablespoons unseasoned breadcrumbs
- ½ teaspoon Tabasco sauce (optional)
- 1 ½ teaspoons dry Hidden Valley Original Ranch Salad Dressing and Seasoning Mix

NUTRITIONAL VALUES PER SERVING: 7-8 PIECES	
Calories	233
Fat	13 g
Carbohydrates	24 g
Protein	5 g
Sodium	212 mg
Potassium	215 mg
Phosphorus	86 mg

DIRECTIONS:

1. Whisk together egg, hot sauce, and milk in a bowl. Dry the eggplant slices with paper towels.
2. Combine breadcrumbs, cornstarch, dry ranch salad, and dressing mix in a shallow bowl.
3. Pour oil into a pan and heat it over high heat.
4. Meanwhile, dunk the eggplant sticks in egg mixture. Shaking off excess liquid, dredge in the breadcrumb mixture and place on a plate.
5. When oil is hot, around 365°F, add the breaded eggplant sticks in the pan and cook until golden brown all over, turning occasionally.
6. Remove the fries with a slotted spoon and place on a plate lined with paper towels.

199. FRIED TOFU WITH DIPPING SAUCE

Prep. time: 5 min | Cooking time: 15 min | Servings: 1

INGREDIENTS:

- 3 ounces firm tofu
- ½ clove garlic, minced
- ½ teaspoon sugar
- ¾ teaspoon sesame oil
- 1 tablespoon vegetable oil
- ½ green onion, sliced
- ½ teaspoon red pepper flakes
- 1 teaspoon low-sodium soy sauce

NUTRITIONAL VALUES PER SERVING	
Calories	219
Fat	19 g
Carbohydrates	6 g
Protein	200 g
Sodium	200 mg
Potassium	176 mg
Phosphorus	132 mg

DIRECTIONS:

1. Cut tofu into rectangles. Dry the tofu pieces with paper towels.
2. Pour vegetable oil into a pan and place the pan over medium-low heat. When oil is hot, add tofu slices and cook until golden brown all over, turning occasionally.
3. Remove tofu with a slotted spoon and place on a plate lined with paper towels.
4. Make the dipping sauce by mixing together garlic, sugar, sesame oil, green onion, soy sauce, and red pepper flakes in a bowl.
5. Serve fried tofu with dipping sauce.

200. CHEESE DIP

Prep. time: 10 min | Cooking time: 0 min | Servings: 6

INGREDIENTS:

- ¾ cup cottage cheese
- ½ teaspoon dill
- ½ cup sour cream
- 1 teaspoon Tabasco sauce
- ¼ teaspoon garlic powder
- 1 ½ green onions, chopped into big pieces
- 3 tablespoon crumbled blue cheese

NUTRITIONAL VALUES PER SERVING: 3 TABLESPOONS (WITHOUT SERVING OPTIONS)	
Calories	78
Fat	5 g
Carbohydrates	3 g
Protein	4 g
Sodium	140 mg
Potassium	78 mg
Phosphorus	73 mg

DIRECTIONS:

1. Place cottage cheese, green onion, garlic powder, sour cream, hot sauce, and dill in a blender or food processor and blend until smooth. Blend in the blue cheese.
2. Pour into a bowl and serve with vegetable sticks or low-sodium crackers if desired.

201. CRANBERRY DIP WITH FRESH FRUIT

Prep. time: 15 min | Cooking time: 0 min | Servings: 3

INGREDIENTS:

- 1 ounce sour cream
- A pinch ground nutmeg
- ½ cup chopped pineapple chunks (9 chunks)
- ½ medium pear, cored, peeled, cut into 6 slices
- ⅛ teaspoon lemon juice
- 1 tablespoon whole berry cranberry sauce
- A pinch ground ginger
- ½ medium apple, cored, cut into 6 slices

NUTRITIONAL VALUES PER SERVING: 2 TABLESPOONS DIP WITH 3 PINEAPPLE CHUNKS, (2 SLICES PEAR, AND 2 SLICES APPLE)	
Calories	70
Fat	2 g
Carbohydrates	13 g
Protein	0 g
Sodium	8 mg
Potassium	101 mg
Phosphorus	15 mg

DIRECTIONS:

1. Pour enough water into a pot such that it is about 2 inches in height from the bottom of the pot. Place the pot over high heat and let it start boiling.
2. Place carrots in a steamer basket and place the basket in the pot. Cover the steamer basket and cook for 10 minutes or until soft.
3. Transfer the carrots into a bowl and mash them using a potato masher until the texture you desire is achieved. If you want a smooth texture, you can blend with an immersion blender.
4. Stir in honey, vanilla, ginger, pepper, and chives if using and stir.

202. RAW VEGGIES AND DIP

Prep. time: 5 min | Cooking time: 0 min + chilling time | Servings: 4

INGREDIENTS:

- ¼ cup sour cream
- 1 teaspoon Mrs. Dash onion herb seasoning
- 1 stalk celery, cut into 8 equal pieces
- ½ bell pepper, cut into 4 equal pieces
- ½ carrot, cut into 4 equal pieces
- 4 radishes, trimmed, scrubbed if desired
- ¼ cucumber, cut into 4 equal pieces

NUTRITIONAL VALUES PER SERVING*	
Calories	37
Fat	2 g
Carbohydrates	3 g
Protein	1 g
Sodium	20 mg
Potassium	140 mg
Phosphorus	25 mg

*2 pieces celery and 1 piece each of carrot, cucumber, bell pepper, and radish with 1 tablespoon dip

DIRECTIONS:

1. Mix together sour cream and seasoning in a bowl. Cover the bowl and chill for 1-2 hours.
2. Place the vegetables on a serving platter. Place the dip on the platter and serve.

203. BUFFALO CHICKEN DIP

Prep. time: 5 min | Cooking time: 30 min | Servings: 4

INGREDIENTS:

- 1 ounce cream cheese, softened
- ¼ cup reduced-fat sour cream
- ½ cup cooked, shredded chicken
- ⅛ up bottled roasted red peppers, drained
- 1 teaspoons Tabasco hot pepper sauce

NUTRITIONAL VALUES PER SERVING: ¼ CUP DIP (WITHOUT SERVING OPTIONS)	
Calories	73
Fat	5 g
Carbohydrates	2 g
Protein	5 g
Sodium	66 mg
Potassium	81 mg
Phosphorus	47 mg

DIRECTIONS:

1. Preheat the oven to 350°F.
2. Add red pepper into the small blender jar and blend until smooth. Pour into a baking dish.
3. Add cream cheese, sour cream, and Tabasco sauce into the baking dish and mix until well combined
4. Stir in the chicken and mix until well coated.
5. Bake the dip in the oven for about 30 minutes or until the chicken is heated thoroughly. You can also cook it on low setting in a slow cooker.
6. Serve with vegetable sticks or low-sodium crackers.

204. BEAN DIP

Prep. time: 15 min | Cooking time: 5-6 min | Servings: 8

INGREDIENTS:

- ¼ large red onion, chopped
- ½ red bell pepper, chopped
- ½ green bell pepper, chopped
- 3 tablespoons chopped cilantro
- ½ cup cooked pinto beans
- 1 ¼ cups cooked white hominy beans
- 2 cloves garlic, minced
- 4 ounces low-fat cream cheese
- ⅛ teaspoon chili powder
- Juice of ½ lime
- 4 ounces low-fat cream cheese
- 2 cloves garlic, peeled
- 6 ounces low-fat sour cream
- ½ tablespoon ground cumin

NUTRITIONAL VALUES PER SERVING: 1 ½ INCHES SQUARE PORTION

Calories	58
Fat	4 g
Carbohydrates	4 g
Protein	2 g
Sodium	58 mg
Potassium	64 mg
Phosphorus	31 mg

DIRECTIONS:

1. Place pinto beans, hominy beans, oil, cream cheese, garlic, chili powder, and cumin in a food processor bowl and process until smooth and well combined.
2. Pour into a small square pan (about 6 inches). Spread it evenly.
3. Next spread the sour cream evenly with a spatula.
4. Place a nonstick pan over medium heat. Add bell peppers, remaining garlic, and onion and stir. Add half the garlic and cook for a few minutes until crisp as well as tender. Discard any liquid from the pan.
5. Add lime juice and stir. Scatter the vegetable mixture over the sour cream and serve. You can serve it chilled or at room temperature.

205. HOT CRAB DIP

Prep. time: 5 min | Cooking time: 15 min | Servings: 5

INGREDIENTS:

- 4 ounces cream cheese, softened at room temperature
- ½ teaspoon lemon juice
- A pinch black pepper
- 1 tablespoon 1% low-fat milk
- ½ tablespoon minced onion
- 1 teaspoon Worcestershire sauce
- A pinch cayenne pepper
- 3 ounces canned crab meat

NUTRITIONAL VALUES PER SERVING: 3 TABLESPOONS (WITHOUT SERVING OPTIONS)

Calories	96
Fat	8 g
Carbohydrates	1 g
Protein	8 g
Sodium	191 mg
Potassium	92 mg
Phosphorus	68 mg

DIRECTIONS:

1. Preheat the oven to 375°F.
2. Combine cream cheese, onion, milk, Worcestershire sauce, cayenne pepper, black pepper, and lemon juice in a bowl.
3. Stir in the crab meat. Transfer the mixture into an oven-safe baking dish.
4. Place the baking dish in the oven and set the timer for 15 minutes.
5. Serve warm with vegetable sticks or low-salt tortilla chips or low-salt crackers.

206. ARTICHOKE DIP

Prep. time: 5 min | Cooking time: 6 min | Servings: 5

INGREDIENTS:

- ½ cup frozen artichoke hearts
- ⅛ cup sour cream
- ½ large clove garlic, minced
- 1 tablespoon cream cheese
- 1 teaspoon hot sauce
- ½ tablespoon parmesan cheese
- ⅛ cup low sodium mayonnaise—refer to the Vegetarian Reuben sandwich for the recipe

NUTRITIONAL VALUES PER SERVING: 2 TABLESPOONS (WITHOUT SERVING OPTIONS)	
Calories	119
Fat	11 g
Carbohydrates	3 g
Protein	2 g
Sodium	106 mg
Potassium	99 mg
Phosphorus	36 mg

DIRECTIONS:

1. Preheat the oven to 375°F.
2. Add artichoke hearts in a pot of water. Place the pot over high heat. When it starts boiling, lower the heat to medium heat and drain off after 6 minutes.
3. Rinse under cold running water.
4. Now cut the artichoke hearts into smaller pieces.
5. Add mayonnaise, cream cheese, garlic, and hot sauce into a bowl and whisk well.
6. Stir in artichoke hearts and spoon the mixture into a baking dish.
7. Sprinkle parmesan cheese on top. Place the baking dish in the oven and set the timer for 30 minutes or until the dip is bubbling.
8. Serve with vegetable sticks or low-sodium crackers or tortilla chips.

207. SEAFOOD DIP

Prep. time: 10 min | Cooking time: 0 min + + chilling time | Servings: 5

INGREDIENTS:

- 4 ounces cream cheese, softened at room temperature
- 2 ounces imitation crabmeat, chopped
- 4 ounces frozen, cooked shrimp, thawed, deveined, peeled, chopped
- ½ unsalted ketchup
- ½ tablespoon lemon juice
- ¼ teaspoon Tabasco sauce
- ¾ tablespoon prepared horseradish
- ½ tablespoon low-sodium Worcestershire sauce
- 15 low-sodium crackers

NUTRITIONAL VALUES PER SERVING: ¼ CUP DIP WITH 3 CRACKERS	
Calories	187
Fat	11 g
Carbohydrates	14 g
Protein	8 g
Sodium	256 mg
Potassium	163 mg
Phosphorus	82 mg

DIRECTIONS:

1. Combine crabmeat and shrimp in a bowl. Cover the bowl and place it in the refrigerator.
2. To make cocktail sauce: Add ketchup, lemon juice, horseradish, and Worcestershire sauce in a small bowl. Whisk cream cheese until creamy. Add the sauce mixture and mix until smooth. Stir in Tabasco sauce.
3. Add the shrimp mixture and mix well. Cover the bowl and chill for 8-9 hours.

208. ONION HERB FLATBREAD CRACKERS WITH PEACHY DIP

Prep. time: 15 min | Cooking time: 7-9 min | Servings: 24

INGREDIENTS:

CRACKERS:
- 4 teaspoons sugar
- ⅔ cup olive oil
- 1 cup water
- 2 egg whites
- 3 ½ cups all-purpose white flour
- 3 tablespoons Mrs. Dash onion and herb seasoning blend

DIP:
- 1 cup nonfat Greek yogurt
- 2 tablespoons yellow mustard
- 6 tablespoons peach preserves or jam

NUTRITIONAL VALUES
PER SERVING: 1 TABLESPOON DIP
WITH 4 CRACKERS

Calories	138
Fat	6 g
Carbohydrates	18 g
Protein	3 g
Sodium	24 mg
Potassium	55 mg
Phosphorus	32 mg

DIRECTIONS:

1. To make dip: Add yogurt, mustard, and peach preserves into a bowl. Mix well. Cover the bowl and chill until use.
2. Preheat the oven to 400°F.
3. To make crackers: Add flour, sugar, and seasoning into a mixing bowl and stir until well combined.
4. Make a cavity in the center of the flour mixture. Pour oil, egg whites, and oil into the cavity and mix well with your hands or you can also use a stand mixer with a dough hook attachment.
5. Mix until you get dough. Knead the dough for 3-4 minutes on a floured area.
6. Make 8 equal portions of the dough.
7. Dust your countertop with some more flour. Place a ball of dough on your countertop and roll the dough until it is a very thin rectangle. Cut into 12 equal crackers.
8. Repeat the same with the remaining dough balls. Take 2 large baking sheets and place the crackers on the baking sheet. Prick holes on the crackers to avoid rising while baking.
9. Place baking sheets in the oven in batches and bake for 7-9 minutes or until light brown and crisp.
10. Cool completely and transfer into an airtight container. Serve with peachy dip.

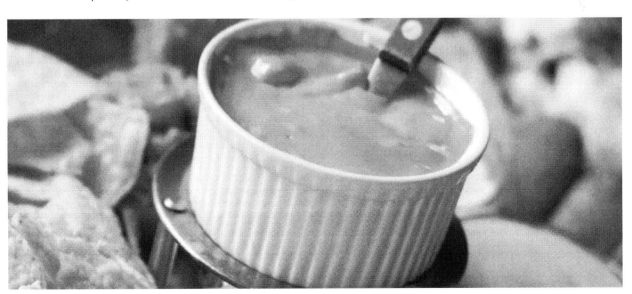

209. PUMPKIN PEPPER HUMMUS

Prep. time: 10 min I Cooking time: 1 hour and 15 min I Servings: 4-5

INGREDIENTS:

- 2 cups canned pumpkin
- ½ teaspoon garlic powder
- ¼ teaspoon harissa seasoning
- 2 large red bell peppers
- ½ teaspoon black pepper

NUTRITIONAL VALUES PER SERVING: ½ CUP	
Calories	34
Fat	0.3 g
Carbohydrates	7.8 g
Protein	1.2 g
Sodium	7 mg
Potassium	217 mg
Phosphorus	33.2 mg

DIRECTIONS:

1. Preheat the oven to 375°F. Remove the stem and seeds from the bell peppers and place them in a baking dish. Place the baking dish in the oven and set the timer for an hour.
2. Once roasted, let the bell peppers cool on your countertop for about 15 minutes.
3. Chop into chunks and place it in a blender along with pumpkin and seasonings and blend until smooth. Pour into a bowl. Serve with vegetable sticks or low-salt cracker or tortilla chips.

210. LEMON PEPPER HUMMUS

Prep. time: 8-10 min I Cooking time: 5 min I Servings: 5

INGREDIENTS:

- 1 can (15 ounces) chickpeas, drained, rinsed
- Juice of ½ lemon
- A pinch garlic powder
- 3 tablespoons olive oil
- ½ teaspoon salt-free lemon pepper seasoning

NUTRITIONAL VALUES PER SERVING: ¼ CUP	
Calories	128
Fat	8 g
Carbohydrates	11 g
Protein	3 g
Sodium	98 mg
Potassium	60 mg
Phosphorus	38 mg

DIRECTIONS:

1. Add chickpeas, 1 ½ tablespoons oil, lemon pepper, lemon juice, and garlic powder into a blender and blend until smooth or the texture you desire is achieved. Add a little water if required while blending. Pour into a bowl. Drizzle remaining oil on top.
2. Serve with vegetable sticks, pita, pita chips, or low-salt cracker or tortilla chips.

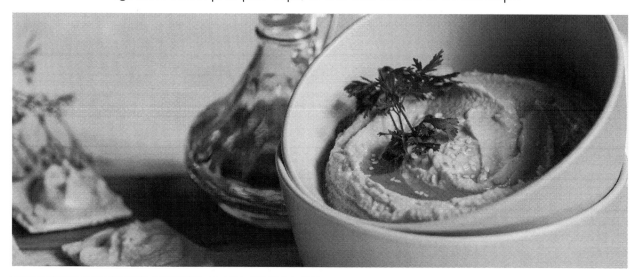

211. CUMIN SWEET POTATO SHOESTRING FRIES

Prep. time: 10 min + soaking time | Cooking time: 20-30 min | Servings: 2

INGREDIENTS:

- ½ teaspoon ground cumin
- A pinch salt
- ½ teaspoon olive oil
- ⅛ teaspoon black pepper
- 1 medium sweet potato, peeled, cut into ¼ inch thick, long slices

NUTRITIONAL VALUES PER SERVING: ½ THE RECIPE	
Calories	65
Fat	1 g
Carbohydrates	13 g
Protein	1 g
Sodium	109 mg
Potassium	153 mg
Phosphorus	33 mg

DIRECTIONS:

1. Place sweet potatoes in a bowl of water for 8-9 hours. Change the water after about 4 hours of soaking. Drain well. Preheat the oven to 425°F.
2. Dry the potatoes by patting with paper towels and place them in a resealable bag.
3. Sprinkle the spices over the sweet potatoes and drizzle oil. Seal the bag and shake well.
4. Spread the sweet potatoes on a baking sheet and place it in the oven. Set the timer for 20 minutes or until brown and crisp.

212. CUCUMBER CUPS STUFFED WITH BUFFALO CHICKEN SALAD

Prep. time: 15 min | Cooking time: 0 min + chilling time | Servings: 4

INGREDIENTS:

- ¼ teaspoon black pepper
- ¼ teaspoon Italian seasoning
- 1 tablespoon hot sauce
- ⅛ cup blue cheese crumbs
- ½ tablespoon chopped garlic
- ½ teaspoon smoked paprika
- ½ teaspoon cayenne pepper
- ¼ cup Kraft mayonnaise
- 1 tablespoon chopped chives
- 1 ½ cups diced or shredded chicken breast
- Chopped fresh parsley to garnish
- 1 tablespoon fresh lemon juice
- 1 large (15 inches long) seedless cucumber, cut into 1 inch thick, round slices

NUTRITIONAL VALUES PER SERVING: ¼ OF THE RECIPE	
Calories	155
Fat	13 g
Carbohydrates	4 g
Protein	18 g
Sodium	252 mg
Potassium	283 mg
Phosphorus	159 mg

DIRECTIONS:

1. Add hot sauce, blue cheese, mayonnaise, lemon juice, chives, and seasonings in a bowl and mix well.
2. Add chicken and stir. Cover the bowl and place it in the refrigerator for 30-40 minutes.
3. Meanwhile, scoop out a little of the pulp from the center of the cucumber slices, making sure to keep the base intact.
4. Place heaping spoonfuls of the salad over the cucumber slices. Sprinkle parsley on top and serve.

213. BEEF PINWHEELS

Prep. time: 10 min | Cooking time: 0 min | Servings: 2

INGREDIENTS:

- 1 flour tortilla (6 inches)
- 4 cucumber slices
- 2.5 ounces roast beef, cooked
- ⅛ bell pepper of any color, cut into strips
- 1 romaine lettuce leaf, shredded
- 1 tablespoon whipped cream cheese
- 2 tablespoons chopped red onion
- ½ teaspoon Mrs. Dash herb seasoning blend

NUTRITIONAL VALUES PER SERVING: 3 PIECES	
Calories	129
Fat	5 g
Carbohydrates	9 g
Protein	12 g
Sodium	139.5 mg
Potassium	224 mg
Phosphorus	126.5 mg

DIRECTIONS:

1. Place the tortilla on your cutting board and spread cream cheese all over it.
2. Scatter beef, bell pepper, lettuce, onion, and cucumber slices over the tortilla. Season with Mrs. Dash herb seasoning. Roll the tortilla along with the filling and place with its seam side facing down.
3. Cut into 1 inch pieces and place on a serving platter. Serve.

214. ZUCCHINI TORTILLA BITES

Prep. time: 20 min | Cooking time: 20 min | Servings: 2

INGREDIENTS:

- 1 corn tortilla, cut into 4 wedges
- ½ zucchini
- Juice of ½ lime
- Zest of ½ lime, grated
- A pinch red pepper flakes
- 1 teaspoon vegetable oil
- ½ cup arugula
- 1 tablespoon chopped cilantro

NUTRITIONAL VALUES PER SERVING: 2 BITES	
Calories	66
Fat	2.9 g
Carbohydrates	9.8 g
Protein	1.9 g
Sodium	13.8 mg
Potassium	271.2 mg
Phosphorus	74.2 mg

DIRECTIONS:

1. Preheat the oven to 375°F.
2. Place the tortilla wedges on a baking sheet and bake for 8-10 minutes until crisp.
3. In the meantime, peel the zucchini into ribbons.
4. Add oil into a skillet. Place the skillet over medium-high heat. When oil is hot, add arugula, zucchini, lime juice, and lime zest and cook until dry.
5. Divide the vegetables among the tortilla triangles. Garnish with cilantro and red pepper flakes and serve.

215. DEVILED EGGS

Prep. time: 5 min | Cooking time: 0 min | Servings: 1

INGREDIENTS:

NUTRITIONAL VALUES	
PER SERVING: ½ THE RECIPE	
Calories	137
Fat	11 g
Carbohydrates	1 g
Protein	6 g
Sodium	176 mg
Potassium	66 mg
Phosphorus	94 mg

- 1 large egg
- ¼ teaspoon dry mustard
- ¼ teaspoon black pepper
- 1 teaspoon canned pimento
- 1 tablespoon mayonnaise
- A pinch paprika

DIRECTIONS:

1. Place egg in a saucepan. Pour enough water to cover the egg.
2. Place the saucepan over medium-high heat. Cover the pot and let it start boiling. Let it boil for 2-3 minutes (rolling boil).
3. Turn off the heat and do not uncover for 15 minutes. Drain off the hot water and immerse the egg in cold water.
4. When the egg cools, peel it and cut into 2 halves along the length.
5. Scoop out the yolk and place in a bowl. Add mustard, pepper, and mayonnaise.
6. Spoon the yolk mixture into the cavity of the eggs. Garnish with paprika and serve.

216. TURKEY BACON, EGG, AND CHEESE DEVILED EGGS

Prep. time: 5 min | Cooking time: 10-12 min | Servings: 3

INGREDIENTS:

NUTRITIONAL VALUES	
PER SERVING	
Calories	116
Fat	8.3 g
Carbohydrates	1.9 g
Protein	8.1 g
Sodium	255.4 mg
Potassium	106.1 mg
Phosphorus	120.7 mg

- 1 tablespoon chopped spring onion or scallion
- 1 ½ tablespoons light mayonnaise
- 3 large eggs
- 1 slice cooked turkey bacon
- ½ tablespoon mustard
- ⅛ teaspoon pepper
- ½ tablespoon reduced- fat sharp cheddar cheese

DIRECTIONS:

1. Place eggs in a saucepan. Pour enough water to cover the eggs.
2. Place the saucepan over medium-high heat. Cover the pot and let it start boiling. Let it boil for 2-3 minutes (rolling boil).
3. Turn off the heat and do not uncover for 15 minutes. Drain off the hot water and immerse the egg in cold water. When the eggs cool, peel and cut into 2 halves along the length.
4. Scoop out the yolks and place in a bowl. Add mustard, pepper, half the bacon, cheese, and mayonnaise. Stir well.
5. Spoon the yolk mixture into the cavity of the eggs. Garnish with remaining bacon and green onion and serve.

217. SPICE RUBBED CORN

Prep. time: 5 min | Cooking time: 20 min | Servings: 4

INGREDIENTS:

- 2 corn cobs, husked, cut each into 2 halves
- ½ teaspoon curry powder
- ½ teaspoon smoked paprika
- Olive oil to brush
- ½ teaspoon ground cumin
- ½ teaspoon unsalted garlic powder

NUTRITIONAL VALUES PER SERVING: 3 PIECES	
Calories	70
Fat	2.1 g
Carbohydrates	12.9 g
Protein	2.2 g
Sodium	1 mg
Potassium	141 mg
Phosphorus	49 mg

DIRECTIONS:

1. Combine curry powder, paprika, cumin, and garlic powder in a bowl.
2. Brush oil over the corn cob halves. Sprinkle the spice mixture all over the cobs.
3. Take a large sheet of heavy duty foil and place the corn cobs in the center of the foil sheet.
4. Wrap up the corn but leave sufficient space between the foil and corn cobs for the steam to move around.
5. Preheat a grill to medium heat. Place the corn packet on the gill and grill for 10 minutes. Turn the packet over and grill for another 10 minutes.

218. CHEX MIX

Prep. time: 10 min | Cooking time: 35-45 min | Servings: 6

INGREDIENTS:

- ½ cup chopped dried apples
- 1 cup Rice Chex cereal
- 1 ½ cups Cinnamon Chex cereal
- 1 cup Corn Chex cereal
- 1 cup Shredded Wheat Bite-size cereal
- ½ cup dried cranberries, sweetened
- ¼ cup sugar
- ⅛ cup liquid egg whites
- 1 tablespoon apple juice
- ½ tablespoon sesame seeds
- ½ teaspoon cinnamon

NUTRITIONAL VALUES PER SERVING: ¾ CUP	
Calories	214
Fat	2 g
Carbohydrates	46 g
Protein	3 g
Sodium	159 mg
Potassium	118 mg
Phosphorus	67 mg

DIRECTIONS:

1. Preheat the oven to 300°F.
2. Grease a baking dish with cooking spray.
3. Add all the cereals, apple, and cranberries into a bowl and toss well.
4. Add whites, apple juice, sugar, and cinnamon into another bowl and beat well with an electric hand mixer until frothy.
5. Pour over the cereal mixture and stir until well coated.
6. Scatter sesame seeds and toss well. Spoon the mixture into the baking dish. Spread it all over the dish.
7. Place the baking dish in the oven and set the timer for about 30-45 minutes or until light brown and crisp. Stir every 12-15 minutes.
8. Let it cool to room temperature. Transfer into an airtight container and store until use.

219. SPICY PRETZELS

Prep. time: 5 min | Cooking time: 50-60 min | Servings: 16

INGREDIENTS:

- ½ bag (from a 32 ounces bag) unsalted bite-size pretzels (preferably bite size braided twist pretzels)
- 1 tablespoon Hidden Valley Ranch Salad Dressing and

Seasoning mix
- 1 ½ tablespoons dried dill weed
- ½ cup canola oil
- 1 ½ teaspoons garlic powder

NUTRITIONAL VALUES
PER SERVING: 1 OUNCE
(ABOUT 7-8 BITE SIZE PRETZELS)

Calories	184
Fat	8 g
Carbohydrates	22 g
Protein	2 g
Sodium	60 mg
Potassium	43 mg
Phosphorus	28 mg

DIRECTIONS:

1. Preheat the oven to 175°F.
2. Scatter the pretzels on a large baking sheet. If you are unable to find bite-size pretzels, you can take larger pretzels and break them into bite-size pieces.
3. Combine garlic powder and dill in a bowl.
4. Remove half of this mixture into another bowl. To this, add salad dressing mix and 6 tablespoons oil and mix well. Drizzle this mixture over the pretzels and mix well using your hands to coat the pretzels evenly.
5. Once the pretzels are well coated, spread them evenly on the baking sheet.
6. Place the baking sheet in the oven and set the timer for an hour. Turn the pretzels over every 15 minutes.
7. Take out the baking sheet from the oven. Once they cool completely, sprinkle the remaining garlic powder mixture over the pretzels. Drizzle remaining oil and toss well. Serve.
8. Store leftovers in an airtight container.

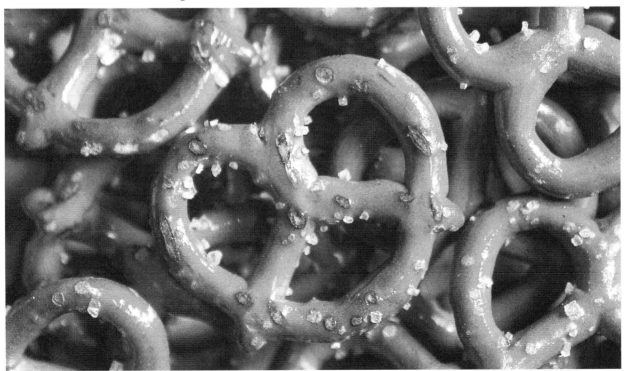

220. FLOUR TORTILLA CHIPS

Prep. time: 5 min I Cooking time: 15 min I Servings: 3

INGREDIENTS:

- ¼ cup canola oil or more if required
- 3 flour tortillas (6 inches each), cut each into 8 wedges

NUTRITIONAL VALUES PER SERVING: 8 CHIPS	
Calories	163
Fat	11 g
Carbohydrates	14 g
Protein	2 g
Sodium	200 mg
Potassium	41 mg
Phosphorus	54 mg

DIRECTIONS:

1. Pour oil into a skillet and heat over medium heat. The oil in the skillet should be at least ¼ inch in height from the bottom of the skillet so add more oil if required.
2. When the oil is hot, about 360°F, drop the tortilla pieces in the oil. Cook until golden brown, turning occasionally. Remove chips with a slotted spoon and place on a plate lined with paper towels. Transfer into an airtight container.

221. SWEET AND SPICY TORTILLA CHIPS

Prep. time: 5 min I Cooking time: 8-10 min I Servings: 4

INGREDIENTS:

- 2 tablespoons butter, melted
- ¼ teaspoon chili powder
- ¼ teaspoon ground cumin
- ½ teaspoon brown sugar
- ¼ teaspoon ground cumin
- 3 flour tortillas (6 inches each), cut each into 8 wedges

NUTRITIONAL VALUES PER SERVING: 6 CHIPS	
Calories	115
Fat	7 g
Carbohydrates	11 g
Protein	2 g
Sodium	156 mg
Potassium	42 mg
Phosphorus	44 mg

DIRECTIONS:

1. Preheat the oven to 425°F. Grease a baking sheet by spraying with cooking spray.
2. Place the tortilla wedges on the baking sheet without overlapping.
3. Combine butter, spices, and brown sugar in a bowl. Brush this mixture over the tortilla wedges.
4. Place the baking sheet in the oven and bake until crisp and brown. Cool completely.
5. Transfer into an airtight container.

222. CRUNCHY MUNCHY SNACK MIX

Prep. time: 5 min | Cooking time: 45 min | Servings: 10

INGREDIENTS:

- 2 cups Ralston Purina Rice Chex cereal
- 1 ½ cups bite size oyster crackers
- 1 cup Kellogg's Crispex cereal
- ½ cup unsalted pretzel twists
- ½ tablespoon chili powder
- ¼ teaspoon garlic powder
- ¾ teaspoon Worcestershire sauce
- 2 ½ tablespoons unsalted, trans-fat free margarine
- ⅛ teaspoon ground cumin
- A pinch cayenne pepper
- ¾ teaspoon lemon juice

NUTRITIONAL VALUES PER SERVING: ½ CUP	
Calories	92
Fat	3 g
Carbohydrates	14 g
Protein	1 g
Sodium	127 mg
Potassium	37 mg
Phosphorus	16 mg

DIRECTIONS:

1. Preheat the oven to 250°F.
2. Combine spices, lemon juice, and Worcestershire sauce. Stir in cereals, pretzels, and crackers.
3. Spread the mixture on a baking sheet. Place the baking sheet in the oven and set the timer for 45 minutes. Stir the mixture every 15 minutes, making sure to spread it evenly.
4. Transfer into an airtight container on cooling.

223. HERBED BISCUITS

Prep. time: 10-12 min | Cooking time: 10 min | Servings: 6

INGREDIENTS:

- ¾ cup + ⅛ cup all-purpose flour
- ¼ teaspoon baking soda
- ½ teaspoon cream of tartar
- 2 tablespoons mayonnaise
- 1 ½ tablespoons chopped chives or any herbs of your choice
- ⅓ cup skim milk

NUTRITIONAL VALUES PER SERVING: 1 BISCUIT	
Calories	109
Fat	4 g
Carbohydrates	15 g
Protein	3 g
Sodium	88 mg
Potassium	85 mg
Phosphorus	34 mg

DIRECTIONS:

1. Preheat the oven to 400°F.
2. Grease a baking sheet by spraying with cooking spray.
3. Add all the dry ingredients into a bowl, i.e. flour, baking soda, and cream of tartar and stir.
4. Add mayonnaise and stir using a fork until coarse and sand-like in texture.
5. Scatter the herbs over the mixture. Pour milk and stir until well-incorporated.
6. Scoop out heaping tablespoonfuls of the batter and place on the baking sheet. Repeat with all the batter making sure to leave a gap between the biscuits.
7. Place the baking sheet in the oven and set the timer for 10 minutes. Cook until light brown on top.
8. Cool completely and store in an airtight container in the refrigerator.

224. SUGAR AND SPICE POPCORN

Prep. time: 5 min | Cooking time: 3 min | Servings: 2

INGREDIENTS:

NUTRITIONAL VALUES PER SERVING: 2 CUPS	
Calories	120
Fat	7 g
Carbohydrates	12 g
Protein	2 g
Sodium	2 mg
Potassium	56 mg
Phosphorus	60 mg

- 2 cups air-popped popcorn (freshly popped)
- 1 tablespoon sugar
- ⅛ teaspoon ground nutmeg
- 1 tablespoon unsalted butter
- ¼ teaspoon ground cinnamon

DIRECTIONS:

1. Add butter, spices and sugar into a saucepan. Place the saucepan over medium heat. Stir until sugar melts. Turn off the heat.
2. Place popcorn in a bowl. Pour the butter mixture over the popcorn. Toss well and serve right away.

225. HOLIDAY CHEESE BALLS

Prep. time: 10 min | Cooking time: 0 min + chilling time | Servings: 6

INGREDIENTS:

NUTRITIONAL VALUES PER SERVING: 1 CHEESE BALL (WITHOUT SERVING OPTIONS)	
Calories	140
Fat	13 g
Carbohydrates	4 g
Protein	2 g
Sodium	131 mg
Potassium	55 mg
Phosphorus	32 mg

- 4 ounces cream cheese, softened
- 3 tablespoons finely ground walnuts
- ½ teaspoon onion powder
- 2 tablespoons Catalina or Russian salad dressing

DIRECTIONS:

1. Add cream cheese, onion powder, and salad dressing into a bowl and stir until well combined. Chill for 30-40 minutes. Make 6 equal portions of the mixture and shape into balls.
2. Dredge cheese balls in ground walnuts and place on a plate. Wrap each in cling wrap and chill until use. You can serve the cheese balls as it is or with low-salt crackers or sliced apple if desired.

226. FESTIVE PINEAPPLE CHEESE BALL

Prep. time: 10 min | Cooking time: 0 min + chilling time | Servings: 12

INGREDIENTS:

NUTRITIONAL VALUES PER SERVING: 1 CHEESE BALL	
Calories	95
Fat	10 g
Carbohydrates	4 g
Protein	2 g
Sodium	93 mg
Potassium	65 mg
Phosphorus	32 mg

- 12 ounces cream cheese, softened to room temperature
- ¼ cup chopped green bell pepper
- 10 ounces canned crushed pineapple
- ¼ teaspoon garlic powder

DIRECTIONS:

1. Combine cream cheese, bell pepper, pineapple, and garlic powder in a bowl.
2. Make 12 equal portions of the mixture and shape into balls.
3. Keep the balls wrapped in wax paper and place it in the refrigerator for 8-9 hours.

227. FIESTA ROLL-UPS

Prep. time: 10 min | Cooking time: 0 min + chilling time | Servings: 6

INGREDIENTS:

- 2 ounces canned chopped green chilies
- ¼ teaspoon ground cumin
- 2 tablespoons thinly sliced green onion
- 3 flour tortillas (8 inches each)
- ¼ teaspoon garlic powder
- ¼ teaspoon chili powder
- 4 ounces cream cheese

NUTRITIONAL VALUES PER SERVING: 4 PIECES	
Calories	148
Fat	8 g
Carbohydrates	16 g
Protein	3 g
Sodium	260 mg
Potassium	73 mg
Phosphorus	52 mg

DIRECTIONS:

1. Add green chilies, cream cheese, green onion, and spices into a bowl and stir well.
2. Spread ⅓ of the cream cheese mixture all over each tortilla, except the edges.
3. Roll the tortillas starting from one of the edges right to its opposite edge and place with its seam side facing down on a plate. Fasten with toothpicks.
4. Cover the plate with cling wrap and chill for a couple of hours.
5. Cut into 1 inch pieces and serve.

228. CORN AND CHEESE BALLS

Prep. time: 15 min | Cooking time: 10-12 min | Servings: 4

INGREDIENTS:

- 1 cup frozen yellow corn, thawed
- 1 tablespoon chopped cilantro
- 2 slices white bread
- ½ teaspoon chili powder
- ½ teaspoon ground coriander
- ½ teaspoon ground cumin
- ⅛ teaspoon salt
- ½ green chili, minced
- ¼ cup cottage cheese
- ¼ cup all-purpose white flour
- 1 ½ cups vegetable oil

NUTRITIONAL VALUES PER SERVING: 4 CHEESE BALLS	
Calories	253
Fat	13 g
Carbohydrates	27 g
Protein	7 g
Sodium	287 mg
Potassium	169 mg
Phosphorus	86 mg

DIRECTIONS:

1. Add corn and green chilies into a bowl and stir.
2. Add some water into a bowl. Dip the bread slices in it for 10-15 seconds. Squeeze out as much water as possible from the bread slices.
3. Add bread into the corn mixture. Mix well. Add cheese, flour, cilantro, salt, and the spices into a bowl and mix well. Divide the mixture into 16 equal portions and shape into balls.
4. Pour oil into a small deep pan and place with oil over medium heat. When the oil is heated to around 360°F but not smoking, carefully place 4-5 balls in the pan. Cook until golden brown all over. Remove balls with a slotted spoon and place on a plate lined with paper towels.
5. Fry the remaining balls in a similar manner. Serve.

229. TURKEY PINWHEEL SANDWICHES

Prep. time: 15 min | Cooking time: 0 min | Servings: 4

INGREDIENTS:

- 2 roasted red peppers, cut into thin strips
- 4 ounces thinly sliced deli turkey
- 2 cups salad mix greens
- 6 tablespoons whipped cream cheese
- 2 tortilla wraps (10 inches each)

NUTRITIONAL VALUES PER SERVING: 3 PIECES	
Calories	172
Fat	9 g
Carbohydrates	14 g
Protein	9 g
Sodium	440 mg
Potassium	270 mg
Phosphorus	119 mg

DIRECTIONS:

1. Spread 3 tablespoons of whipped cream cheese on each tortilla.
2. Divide the salad greens and turkey slices equally and spread it evenly,
3. Divide the red pepper equally and scatter over the turkey slices.
4. Start rolling from one of the sides and reach up to the other end.
5. Place the rolled tortillas on your cutting board. Fasten with toothpicks.
6. Cut each of the tortillas into 6 slices and serve.

230. SWEET 'N' SOUR MEATBALLS

Prep. time: 12-15 min | Cooking time: 15 min | Servings: 6

INGREDIENTS:

MEATBALLS:
- ½ pound ground turkey (7% fat)
- ⅛ cup unseasoned breadcrumbs
- ½ teaspoon garlic powder
- 2 tablespoons canola oil
- 1 tablespoon minced onion
- ¼ teaspoon pepper
- 1 small egg

SAUCE:
- 2 tablespoons Heinz bottled chili sauce
- 3 ounces grape jelly

NUTRITIONAL VALUES PER SERVING: 4 MEATBALLS	
Calories	127
Fat	4 g
Carbohydrates	14 g
Protein	9 g
Sodium	129 mg
Potassium	148 mg
Phosphorus	89 mg

DIRECTIONS:

1. Add turkey, breadcrumbs, onion, egg, and spices into a bowl and mix until well incorporated.
2. Divide the mixture into 24 equal portions and form balls of each portion.
3. Pour oil into a large skillet and let the pan heat over medium heat. When oil is hot, place the meatballs in the pan and cook until brown on the outside and cooked through inside.
4. Transfer the meatballs into a shallow bowl.
5. Place chili sauce and grape jelly in a microwave safe bowl. Drizzle the sauce over the meatballs. Insert a toothpick in each meatball and serve.

231. CHICKEN PARMESAN MEATBALLS

Prep. time: 15 min | Cooking time: 15 min | Servings: 5

INGREDIENTS:

- ½ pound ground chicken
- 1 ½ tablespoons breadcrumbs
- 4 ounces pizza sauce
- ⅛ teaspoon onion powder
- ⅛ teaspoon Italian seasoning
- ⅛ teaspoon garlic powder
- 1 small egg
- ½ tablespoon grated parmesan cheese
- ¼ cup shredded mozzarella cheese

NUTRITIONAL VALUES PER SERVING: 3 MEATBALLS	
Calories	114
Fat	6 g
Carbohydrates	4 g
Protein	11 g
Sodium	223 mg
Potassium	350 mg
Phosphorus	132 mg

DIRECTIONS:

1. Preheat the oven to 375°F. Grease a baking sheet by spraying with cooking spray.
2. Add chicken, breadcrumbs, 1 tablespoon pizza sauce, egg, parmesan cheese, and spices into a bowl and mix until well-combined.
3. Divide the mixture into 15 equal portions and shape them into balls. Place them on the baking sheet. Place the baking sheet in the oven and set the timer for 15 minutes.
4. Spoon about an ounce of pizza sauce on the bottom of a baking dish. Place the meatballs in the baking dish. Spoon the rest of the pizza sauce over the meatballs. Scatter mozzarella cheese on top.
5. Bake for a few more minutes until the cheese melts. Insert toothpicks in each meatball and serve.

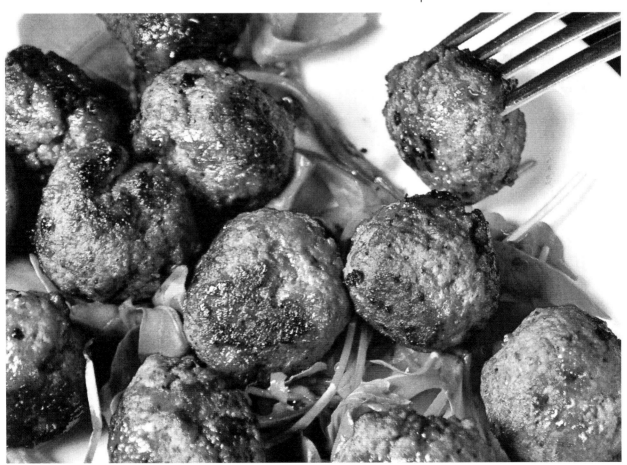

232. CHIPOTLE WINGS

Prep. time: 5 min | Cooking time: 20-25 min | Servings: 2

INGREDIENTS:

- 8 chicken wings or ½ pound large chicken wings cut into 8 pieces
- ¾ tablespoon diced chipotle peppers in adobo sauce
- 2 tablespoons unsalted butter, slightly melted
- ½ tablespoon chopped chives
- 2 tablespoons honey
- ½ teaspoon pepper

NUTRITIONAL VALUES PER SERVING: 4 WINGS	
Calories	384
Fat	26 g
Carbohydrates	18 g
Protein	20 g
Sodium	99 mg
Potassium	266 mg
Phosphorus	146 mg

DIRECTIONS:

1. Preheat the oven to 375°F. Grease a baking sheet by spraying with cooking spray.
2. Place the chicken wings on the baking sheet. Spray the top of the chicken with cooking spray and place it in the oven.
3. Set the timer for 20 minutes. Bake until the internal temperature of the chicken in the thickest part of the meat shows 165°F on a meat thermometer.
4. Combine chipotle peppers, butter, chives, honey, and pepper in a bowl. Add the chicken wings into the bowl and mix until the wings are well-coated with the sauce.

233. HUNGARIAN SOUR CHERRY SOUP

Prep. time: 5 min | Cooking time: 15 min | Servings: 2

INGREDIENTS:

- ¾ cup pitted fresh cherries
- 3 tablespoons sugar
- ½ tablespoon all-purpose flour
- 1 ½ cups water
- A tiny pinch salt
- ¼ cup reduced-fat sour cream

NUTRITIONAL VALUES PER SERVING: 1 CUP	
Calories	144
Fat	4 g
Carbohydrates	25 g
Protein	2 g
Sodium	57 mg
Potassium	144 mg
Phosphorus	40 mg

DIRECTIONS:

1. Cook cherries, sugar, water, and salt in a saucepan over low heat. Take out a tablespoon of the cooked liquid and keep it aside to garnish. Take out another 2 tablespoons of the cooked liquid and place in a bowl. Let it cool for a few minutes.
2. Add flour and sour cream into the bowl of cooled liquid and whisk well. Pour into the saucepan. Whisk well and continue cooking over low heat until slightly thick.
3. Turn off the heat and divide into 2 bowls.
4. Drizzle the retained liquid on top in each bowl. Swirl lightly and serve.

234. CRISPY CAULIFLOWER PHYLLO CUPS

Prep. time: 15 min | Cooking time: 20 min | Servings: 8

INGREDIENTS:

- 1 egg, beaten
- 2 ⅔ tablespoons shredded cheddar cheese
- 2 ⅔ tablespoons shredded, low-sodium Swiss cheese
- ⅔ tablespoon butter
- ½ cup diced, cooked cauliflower, drained
- ⅔ tablespoon diced jalapeño
- ⅓ tablespoon chopped

- parsley + extra to garnish
- 1 phyllo sheet
- 1 ⅓ slices bacon, natural, uncured, diced
- 1 ⅓ tablespoons minced onion
- Red pepper flakes to taste
- Black pepper to taste + extra to garnish

NUTRITIONAL VALUES PER SERVING: 1 CUP	
Calories	68
Fat	5 g
Carbohydrates	2 g
Protein	3 g
Sodium	107 mg
Potassium	42 mg
Phosphorus	49 mg

DIRECTIONS:

1. Preheat the oven to 375°F. Grease a mini muffin pan with some cooking spray.
2. Spray some oil into a pan and place the pan over medium heat. Add egg and stir often and cook until the eggs are soft cooked. Transfer egg into a bowl. Place the skillet back over heat. Add butter. When butter melts, add bacon and cook until light brown. Stir in cauliflower, onion, red pepper flakes, and jalapeño and cook for a couple of minutes until the onion is soft.
3. Add parsley and pepper and mix well. Turn off the heat. Add scrambled egg, cheddar, and Swiss cheese and mix well. Cut the phyllo sheet into 3 equal pieces. Stack them together. Now cut this stack into 8 equal square pieces. Separate the squares and place one in each of 8 mini muffin cups.
4. Press it onto the bottom of the muffin cups. Divide the egg mixture among the muffin cups.
5. Place the muffin pan on the bottom rack in the oven. Bake until the edges of the phyllo sheets turn light golden brown. Switch off the oven. Let it remain in the oven for 3 minutes.
6. Sprinkle pepper and parsley on top and serve.

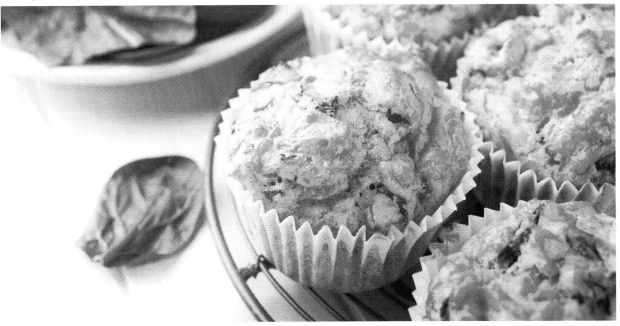

235. CHILLED CUCUMBER SOUP

Prep. time: 10 min | Cooking time: 0 min + chilling time | Servings: 10

INGREDIENTS:

- 4 medium cucumbers, peeled, deseeded, chopped
- 2 green onions, chopped
- ¼ cup fresh dill + extra to garnish
- ⅔ cup chopped sweet white onion
- ½ cup fresh mint leaves
- 1 ⅓ cups water
- ⅔ cup sour cream
- ½ teaspoon salt
- 4 tablespoons lemon juice
- 1 cup half and half creamer
- 1 teaspoon pepper

NUTRITIONAL VALUES PER SERVING: ¾ CUP	
Calories	77
Fat	5 g
Carbohydrates	6 g
Protein	2 g
Sodium	128 mg
Potassium	258 mg
Phosphorus	68 mg

DIRECTIONS:

1. Place cucumber, green onion, dill, mint, onion, water, sour cream, salt, lemon juice, half and half, and pepper into a blender. Blend for 30-40 seconds or until smooth. Pour into a large bowl.
2. Cover the bowl and chill for a few hours. Ladle into soup bowls. Decorate with dill sprigs and serve.

236. THAI PUMPKIN SOUP

Prep. time: 5 min | Cooking time: 30 min | Servings: 3-4

INGREDIENTS:

- ½ onion, minced
- 1 tablespoon brown sugar
- ⅛ teaspoon salt
- ½ can (from a 15 ounce can) low-fat coconut milk
- ¼ teaspoon ground coriander
- A pinch ground nutmeg
- ½ teaspoon curry powder
- ¼ teaspoon ground cinnamon
- ⅛ teaspoon ground ginger
- ¼ cup chopped cilantro
- 2 small cloves garlic, minced
- 1 cup low-sodium vegetable broth
- ⅛ teaspoon black pepper
- ⅛ cup natural creamy peanut butter
- 1 teaspoon olive oil

NUTRITIONAL VALUES PER SERVING: ¾ CUP	
Calories	139
Fat	9 g
Carbohydrates	14 g
Protein	4 g
Sodium	168 mg
Potassium	368 mg
Phosphorus	75 mg

DIRECTIONS:

1. Pour oil into a saucepan. Place the saucepan over medium heat. When oil is hot, add onion, brown sugar, and garlic and cook until onion turns translucent.
2. Stir in pepper, salt, and broth. Let it start boiling.
3. Lower the heat and cook for about 10-12 minutes.
4. Pour coconut milk and pumpkin puree and stir. Add peanut butter and spices. and mix well. Heat the mixture for about 5 minutes. Turn off the heat.
5. Blend with an immersion blender until smooth.
6. Ladle into soup bowls. Garnish with cilantro and serve.

237. SHRIMP SPREAD WITH CRACKERS

Prep. time: 12 min | Cooking time: 0 min | Servings: 4

INGREDIENTS:

- 2 tablespoons light cream cheese, softened to room temperature
- ½ tablespoon unsalted ketchup
- ½ teaspoon Worcestershire sauce
- 12 matzo cracker miniatures
- 1 ¼ ounces cooked, shelled, minced shrimp
- ⅛ teaspoon Tabasco sauce
- ¼ teaspoon Mrs. Dash herb seasoning blend
- ½ tablespoon chopped parsley

NUTRITIONAL VALUES PER SERVING: 3 CRACKERS WITH 3 TEASPOONS SPREAD

Calories	57
Fat	1 g
Carbohydrates	7 g
Protein	3 g
Sodium	69 mg
Potassium	54 mg
Phosphorus	60 mg

DIRECTIONS:

Combine cream cheese, shrimp, Worcestershire sauce, Tabasco sauce, ketchup, and seasoning in a bowl. Spread a teaspoon of the mixture over each cracker. Sprinkle parsley on top and serve.

238. ITALIAN PHYLLO CUPS

Prep. time: 15 min | Cooking time: 30 min | Servings: 6

INGREDIENTS:

- ¼ cup whole almonds
- ¾ teaspoon chopped garlic
- 1 teaspoon dried basil
- ½ tablespoon lemon juice
- A pinch grilling spice blend, unsalted
- ¾ teaspoon vegetable base
- 4 phyllo sheets
- 4 ounces firm tofu
- ⅛ teaspoon dried oregano
- ⅛ teaspoon dried ground thyme
- A pinch onion powder
- 1 drop Tabasco
- ⅛ teaspoon garlic powder

NUTRITIONAL VALUES PER SERVING: 1 CUP

Calories	94
Fat	4.7 g
Carbohydrates	9.1 g
Protein	4.6 g
Sodium	70.1 mg
Potassium	97.7 mg
Phosphorus	70.2 mg

DIRECTIONS:

1. Boil a small pot of water. When water starts boiling, drop the almonds into the pot.
2. Lower the heat and cook for 15 minutes. Drain well and place almonds in the food processor bowl. Process until finely chopped.
3. Add garlic, herbs, lemon juice, spices, and tofu and process until smooth.
4. Pour into a bowl. Add Tabasco sauce and stir.
5. Preheat the oven to 375°F. Grease a muffin pan with cooking spray.
6. Stack the phyllo sheets, spraying with cooking spray in between the sheets.
7. Cut the stack into 6 equal square pieces.
8. Place the phyllo squares in the muffin cups and press it into the cups.
9. Spoon the tofu mixture into the cups.
10. Place the muffin pan in the oven and set the timer for 10-15 minutes or the edges of the stack start to turn golden brown. Let it cool on your countertop for 5 minutes before serving.

239. HEALTHY CHICKEN NUGGETS

Prep. time: 20 min + chilling and thawing time | Cooking time: 25-30 min | Servings: 4-5

INGREDIENTS:

- ¾ pound chicken breast, cut into 1.5 x 1 inch pieces
- ½ cup all-purpose white flour
- ½ cup crushed cornflakes or unsalted corn chips
- ⅛ teaspoon dried dill
- ⅛ teaspoon garlic powder
- ⅛ teaspoon freshly ground pepper
- 8 ounces low-fat Greek yogurt
- 1 small egg, beaten
- ¼ cup lemon juice
- ⅛ teaspoon dried celery seeds
- ⅛ teaspoon grated lemon peel

NUTRITIONAL VALUES PER SERVING: 5 NUGGETS	
Calories	145
Fat	2.3 g
Carbohydrates	17 g
Protein	13.6 g
Sodium	62.3 mg
Potassium	149.3 mg
Phosphorus	120.3 mg

DIRECTIONS:

1. Combine lemon juice and Greek yogurt in a bowl. Add chicken and mix well. Rub the mixture all over the chicken using your hands.
2. Cover the bowl with cling wrap and let it marinate in the refrigerator for 4-8 hours.
3. Take out the bowl from the refrigerator about an hour before baking so that it comes to room temperature. Preheat the oven to 400°F.
4. Place flour in a shallow bowl. Combine crushed cornflakes and spices in another shallow bowl.
5. Prepare a baking sheet by lining it with parchment paper. Place a rack on the baking sheet.
6. First dredge the chicken nuggets in flour, one at a time. Next, dip in egg. Shaking off excess egg, dredge in the cornflakes mixture and place on the rack.
7. When you are done with breading the chicken nuggets, spray some cooking spray all over the nuggets. Place the baking sheet in the oven, along with the rack and chicken.
8. Set the timer for about 20 minutes or bake until crisp and brown. Serve.

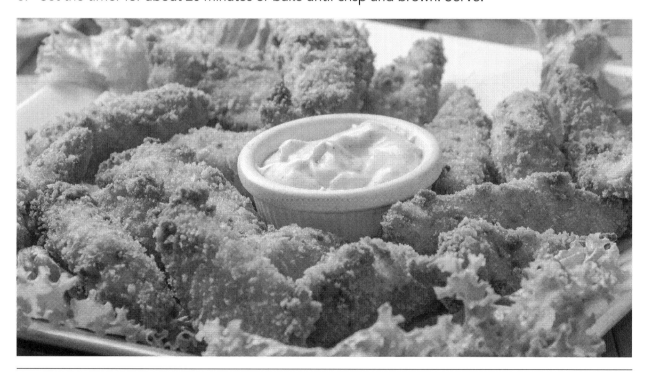

240. APPLE BARS

Prep. time: 15 min | Cooking time: 35-40 min | Servings: 9

INGREDIENTS:

- 1 medium apple, peeled, cored, chopped
- ½ cup granulated sugar
- ½ teaspoon vanilla extract
- ¼ teaspoon salt
- ¼ cup brown sugar
- 1 tablespoon milk
- 6 tablespoons unsalted butter
- ½ cup sour cream
- ½ teaspoon baking soda
- 1 cup all-purpose flour
- ½ teaspoon ground cinnamon
- ½ cup powdered sugar

NUTRITIONAL VALUES PER SERVING	
Calories	246
Fat	11 g
Carbohydrates	35 g
Protein	2 g
Sodium	140 mg
Potassium	72 mg
Phosphorus	27 mg

DIRECTIONS:

1. Preheat the oven to 350°F. Grease a baking pan (about 6 inches) with cooking spray.
2. Place 4 tablespoons unsalted butter and granulated sugar in a bowl. Beat with an electric hand mixer until creamy.
3. Stir in flour, salt, baking soda, vanilla, and sour cream. Make sure the batter is well-combined and smooth.
4. Stir in the apples. Spoon the batter into the baking dish.
5. Combine remaining butter, cinnamon, and brown sugar in a bowl and scatter this mixture over the batter.
6. Place the baking dish in the oven and set the timer for 35-40 minutes.
7. Remove the baking dish from the oven and allow it to cool to room temperature.
8. Cut into 9 equal pieces and serve.

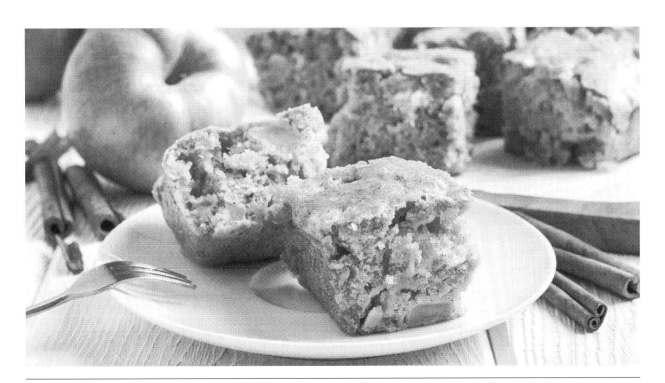

CHAPTER 11
Dessert Recipes

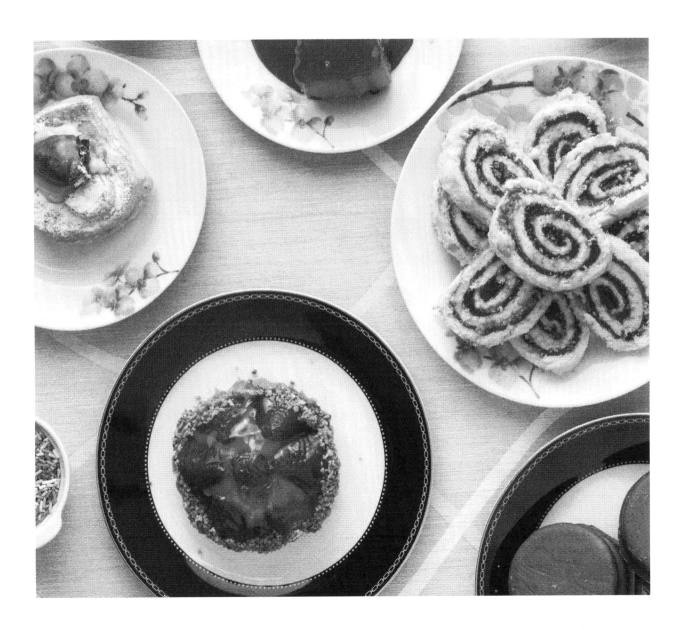

241. FESTIVE FRUIT SALAD

Prep. time: 5 min | Cooking time: 0 min + chilling time | Servings: 5

INGREDIENTS:

- 1 cup cottage cheese
- 1 cup canned pineapple tidbits in juice, drained
- 1.5 ounces lime gelatin mix
- 4 ounces whipped topping

NUTRITIONAL VALUES PER SERVING: ½ CUP	
Calories	179
Fat	3 g
Carbohydrates	29 g
Protein	8 g
Sodium	235 mg
Potassium	90 mg
Phosphorus	88 mg

DIRECTIONS:

1. Place cottage cheese in a bowl. Sprinkle gelatin on top.
2. Combine whipped topping and pineapple in another bowl. Add pineapple mixture into the bowl of cottage cheese and fold gently. Cover the bowl with cling wrap and chill for 8-9 hours. Serve.

242. CARAMEL APPLE SALAD

Prep. time: 10 min | Cooking time: 0 min + chilling time | Servings: 5

INGREDIENTS:

- 1 ½ cups cubed Granny Smith apples, unpeeled
- 4 ounces whipped topping
- 3 tablespoons unsalted, roasted peanuts
- 4 ounces canned crushed
- pineapple with its juice
- ¼ cup butterscotch dessert topping
- ⅛ cup butterscotch baking chips

NUTRITIONAL VALUES PER SERVING: ½ CUP	
Calories	196
Fat	8 g
Carbohydrates	30 g
Protein	1 g
Sodium	37 mg
Potassium	105 mg
Phosphorus	47 mg

DIRECTIONS:

1. Combine pineapple and apple in a bowl.
2. Add whipped topping and butterscotch topping into another bowl and stir well.
3. Add the fruits and stir until well combined. Chill until use.
4. Stir the butterscotch chips and peanuts into the salad just before serving.

243. CARROT PINEAPPLE SALAD

Prep. time: 30 min | Cooking time: 3 min | Servings: 4

INGREDIENTS:

- ½ cup shredded carrots
- 5 ounces apricot nectar
- ½ cup heavy whipping cream
- ½ packet Knox unflavored gelatin
- ¼ cup sugar
- 4 ounces canned crushed pineapple with its juice
- 4 ounces low-fat cream cheese

NUTRITIONAL VALUES PER SERVING: ⅔ CUP	
Calories	214
Fat	10 g
Carbohydrates	27 g
Protein	4 g
Sodium	120 mg
Potassium	205 mg
Phosphorus	62 mg

DIRECTIONS:

1. Place a glass bowl and beaters of the hand mixer in a freezer for about 15 minutes.
2. Heat up ½ cup of apricot nectar in a small saucepan over low heat.
3. Add gelatin into a bowl. Once the apricot nectar is hot, turn off the heat and pour it over the gelatin. Whisk until well-combined.
4. Add remaining apricot nectar and pineapple and stir until well-combined.
5. Add carrots and stir. Keep the bowl in the refrigerator until slightly set.
6. Stir together sugar and cream cheese in a bowl. Take out the chilled bowl and beaters from the freezer and add heavy whipping cream into the bowl.
7. Set the mixer on high speed after fixing the beaters and beat for 2-3 minutes until stiff peaks are formed. Add the whipped cream into the bowl of cottage cheese mixture and fold gently.
8. Add the whipped cream mixture into the bowl of semi-set pineapple mixture and stir with a whisk until well-combined. Chill for 3-4 hours.

244. BLUEBERRY COBBLER

Prep. time: 10 min | Cooking time: 45 min | Servings: 18

INGREDIENTS:

- 8 cups blueberries
- 2 tablespoons cornstarch
- ⅔ cup sugar
- 1 teaspoon ground cinnamon
- 2 tablespoons vegetable oil
- 4 eggs
- ½ teaspoon ground nutmeg
- 1 teaspoon vanilla extract
- 2 teaspoons lemon juice
- 2 cups all-purpose flour
- 2 teaspoons baking powder

NUTRITIONAL VALUES PER SERVING WITHOUT ICE CREAM	
Calories	152
Fat	3 g
Carbohydrates	29 g
Protein	3 g
Sodium	69 mg
Potassium	82 mg
Phosphorus	54 mg

DIRECTIONS:

1. Preheat the oven to 350°F. Grease a large baking dish (13 x 9 inches) with cooking spray.
2. Place blueberries in a bowl. Drizzle lemon juice and toss well. Sprinkle cornstarch over the berries and toss well. Scatter the berries in the baking dish.
3. Add flour, baking powder, sugar, and spices into a bowl and stir.
4. Add oil, eggs, and vanilla into another bowl and whisk well. Add this mixture into the bowl of flour mixture and stir until you get a smooth batter.
5. Drop tablespoonfuls of the dough all over the berries. The berries should be covered in dough. Place the baking dish in the oven and bake for 45-50 minutes or until golden brown on top.
6. Take the baking dish out of the oven and cool until warm.
7. You can serve it as it is or with some ice cream if desired.

245. CREAMY FRUIT SALAD

Prep. time: 25 min | Cooking time: 0 min | Servings: 7

INGREDIENTS:

- 1 medium apple, cored, cubed
- ½ can (from a 15 ounce can) peaches in light syrup, cut into bite size pieces
- ¾ cup halved green grapes
- 1 medium fresh pear, peeled, cored, cubed
- ¾ cup chopped fresh strawberries
- ¼ cup fresh berries of your choice
- 2 ounces low-fat cream cheese
- ½ tablespoon sour cream
- 1 tablespoon sugar
- ½ cup + ⅛ cup heavy whipping cream

NUTRITIONAL VALUES PER SERVING: ¾ CUP	
Calories	174
Fat	10 g
Carbohydrates	19 g
Protein	2 g
Sodium	40 mg
Potassium	175 mg
Phosphorus	43 mg

DIRECTIONS:

1. Place a glass bowl and beaters of the hand mixer in a freezer for about 15 minutes.
2. Combine apple, strawberries, grapes, peaches, and pear in a bowl.
3. Stir together sugar, sour cream, and cream cheese in a bowl.
4. Take out the chilled bowl and beaters from the freezer and add heavy whipping cream into it.
5. Set the mixer on high speed after fixing the beaters and beat for 2-3 minutes until stiff peaks are formed. Add the whipped cream into the bowl of cottage cheese mixture and fold gently.
6. You can serve it now or chill the bowl of fruits as well as cottage cheese mixture until ready to serve.
7. To serve: Combine the fruits and cottage cheese mixture and serve garnished with fresh berries.

246. CRANBERRY RASPBERRY GELATIN SALAD

Prep. time: 30 min | Cooking time: 2 min + chilling time | Servings: 2-3

INGREDIENTS:

- ½ cup frozen raspberries
- ¼ cup chopped celery
- ½ cup ginger ale
- ½ can whole cranberry sauce
- ½ box (from a 0.3 ounce box) raspberry gelatin
- ½ cup water

NUTRITIONAL VALUES PER SERVING: 1 CUP	
Calories	59
Fat	0.2 g
Carbohydrates	14.3 g
Protein	0.6 g
Sodium	21 mg
Potassium	45 mg
Phosphorus	7 mg

DIRECTIONS:

Heat water in a saucepan. Pour into a glass serving bowl. Add cranberry sauce, ginger ale, celery, and raspberries and mix well. Chill for 2-3 hours or until set.

247. FROZEN FRUIT DELIGHT

Prep. time: 10 min | Cooking time: 0 min + freezing time | Servings: 5

INGREDIENTS:

- 3 tablespoons chopped maraschino cherries
- 4 ounces reduced-fat sour cream
- ½ cup sliced strawberries
- A pinch salt
- 4 ounces canned crushed pineapple in juice, drained
- ½ tablespoon lemon juice
- ¼ cup sugar, powdered
- 1 ½ cups Reddi-Wip dairy whipped topping

NUTRITIONAL VALUES PER SERVING: ½ CUP	
Calories	133
Fat	5 g
Carbohydrates	21 g
Protein	1 g
Sodium	59 mg
Potassium	99 mg
Phosphorus	36 mg

DIRECTIONS:

1. Combine fruits, sugar, salt, and sour cream in a bowl.
2. Add whipped topping and fold until well-combined.
3. Spoon the mixture into a freezer safe container and place in the freezer until firm.

248. QUICK FRUIT SORBET

Prep. time: 5 min + freezing time | Cooking time: 0 min | Servings: 4

INGREDIENTS:

- 10 ounces canned crushed pineapple in juice
- 2 plums, pitted, chopped
- ½ cup frozen raspberries, unsweetened

NUTRITIONAL VALUES PER SERVING: ½ CUP	
Calories	71
Fat	0 g
Carbohydrates	17 g
Protein	0 g
Sodium	6 mg
Potassium	170 mg
Phosphorus	13 mg

DIRECTIONS:

1. Freeze the pineapple and juice for about 3 hours.
2. Add the fruits into a food processor and blend until smooth and thick.
3. You can serve right away for a soft serve consistency or pour into a freezer safe container and freeze until firm.

249. STRAWBERRY SORBET

Prep. time: 5 min + freezing time | Cooking time: 0 min | Servings: 8

INGREDIENTS:

- 2 cups frozen or fresh strawberries
- ½ cup water
- 2 tablespoons lemon juice
- 2 ½ cups ice cubes

NUTRITIONAL VALUES PER SERVING: ½ CUP	
Calories	22
Fat	0 g
Carbohydrates	5 g
Protein	0 g
Sodium	2 mg
Potassium	123 mg
Phosphorus	18 mg

DIRECTIONS:

1. Add strawberries, water, lemon juice, and ice cubes into a blender and set on crush mode or blend to the desired consistency.
2. Serve right away. You can serve it as a crush or pour into popsicle molds and freeze until firm.

250. RASPBERRY PEAR SORBET

Prep. time: 5 min | Cooking time: 5-6 min + freezing time | Servings: 3

INGREDIENTS:

- ¼ cup sugar
- ½ cup water
- 3 tablespoons lime juice
- 1 large canned pear half in juice, drained
- ½ tablespoon pear liqueur or vodka (optional)
- 1 cup fresh raspberries + extra to garnish

NUTRITIONAL VALUES PER SERVING: ½ CUP	
Calories	135
Fat	0.4 g
Carbohydrates	31.7 g
Protein	0.9 g
Sodium	2.8 mg
Potassium	168.4 mg
Phosphorus	27.4 mg

DIRECTIONS:

1. To make simple syrup: Combine water and sugar in a saucepan. Place the saucepan over medium heat. When it starts boiling, lower the heat and simmer until sugar dissolves. Stir often. Turn off the heat and let it cool. Pour into a bowl and chill for about an hour.
2. Place raspberries, lime juice, pear, and pear liqueur in a blender and blend until smooth. Pour into the bowl of simple syrup. Mix well and pour into a freezer-safe container and freeze until firm.
3. Take out the frozen mixture and break into pieces and place in the food processor bowl. Process until smooth. Pour it back into the freezer-safe container and freeze until firm.
4. Scoop into bowls. Garnish with raspberries and serve.

251. BLUEBERRY CREAM CONES

Prep. time: 10 min | Cooking time: 0 min + freezing time | Servings: 3

INGREDIENTS:

- 2 ounces cream cheese, softened at room temperature
- ¾ cup whipped topping
- ½ cup + ⅛ fresh or frozen blueberries
- 2 tablespoons blueberry jam or preserves

NUTRITIONAL VALUES PER SERVING	
Calories	177
Fat	9 g
Carbohydrates	21 g
Protein	3 g
Sodium	95 mg
Potassium	81 mg
Phosphorus	40 mg

DIRECTIONS:

1. Beat cream cheese with an electric hand mixer until creamy and light.
2. Add jam and cream cheese and fold gently.
3. Scoop the mixture into the cones. Place in the freezer until you need to serve.

252. VANILLA ICE CREAM

Prep. time: 5 min | Cooking time: 10 min | Servings: 4

INGREDIENTS:

- ½ cup low-cholesterol egg produce
- 1 cup liquid non dairy creamer
- ¼ cup sugar
- ½ tablespoon vanilla extract

NUTRITIONAL VALUES PER SERVING: ½ CUP	
Calories	159
Fat	6 g
Carbohydrates	22 g
Protein	3 g
Sodium	64 mg
Potassium	87 mg
Phosphorus	36 mg

DIRECTIONS:

1. Place egg product and sugar in a microwave safe bowl. Beat until well-combined and sugar dissolves.
2. Add non dairy creamer and stir. Place the bowl in the microwave and cook for about a minute on High or until thick. Stir every 20-25 seconds.
3. Let the mixture cool. Add vanilla and churn the ice cream in an ice cream maker following the manufacturer's instructions.
4. Scoop into bowls and serve right away for a soft serve consistency. If you want firm ice cream, pour into a freezer safe container and freeze until firm.

253. STRAWBERRY MOUSSE

Prep. time: 10 min + freezing time | Cooking time: 0 min | Servings: 3

INGREDIENTS:

- ½ packet unflavored gelatin
- ½ tablespoon lukewarm water
- 5 tablespoons granulated sugar
- ½ cup whipped topping
- 1 ½ cups fresh strawberries
- 6 tablespoons pasteurized egg whites

NUTRITIONAL VALUES PER SERVING: ¾ CUP	
Calories	142
Fat	2 g
Carbohydrates	27 g
Protein	4 g
Sodium	51 mg
Potassium	165 mg
Phosphorus	23 mg

DIRECTIONS:

1. Retain a few slices of strawberries for garnish. Combine water and gelatin in a small bowl.
2. Blend the remaining strawberries in a blender until smooth. Pour into a bowl. Add gelatin mixture and stir. Add 1-2 tablespoons of sugar and stir. Cover the bowl and keep it aside.
3. Beat egg whites in a bowl using an electric hand mixer until soft peaks are formed.
4. Add remaining sugar, a little at a time, while you are beating. Beat until stiff peaks are formed.
5. Add the strawberry mixture and fold gently. Divide the mixture into 3 dessert bowls or glasses.
6. Spoon the whipped topping on top. Decorate with retained strawberry slices and serve.

254. RASPBERRY CHEESECAKE MOUSSE

Prep. time: 15 min | Cooking time: 0 min + chilling time | Servings: 3

INGREDIENTS:

- ½ cup light whipped topping
- 6 tablespoon granular splenda
- ½ teaspoon vanilla extract
- 4 ounces cream cheese, at room temperature
- ½ teaspoon finely grated lemon zest
- ½ cup fresh or frozen raspberries
- Mint sprigs to garnish

NUTRITIONAL VALUES PER SERVING: ½ CUP	
Calories	257
Fat	15 g
Carbohydrates	29 g
Protein	3 g
Sodium	124 mg
Potassium	102 mg
Phosphorus	51 mg

DIRECTIONS:

1. Add cream cheese into a bowl and beat with an electric hand mixer until creamy and light.
2. Add ¼ cup splenda and beat until it dissolves completely. Add vanilla and lemon zest and beat until well combined. Add whipped topping and fold gently.
3. Retain a few raspberries for garnish and add the remaining into a bowl. Crush with a fork. Add 2 tablespoons of splenda and stir. Add into the cream cheese mixture and fold gently.
4. Divide into 3 small glasses. Refrigerate until use.
5. Top with retained raspberries and mint sprigs and serve.

255. SPICY PEACHES

Prep. time: 5 min | Cooking time: 10 min | Servings: 6

INGREDIENTS:

- ½ teaspoon whole cloves
- ¼ teaspoon ground nutmeg
- 1 teaspoon cornstarch
- ⅛ teaspoon ground cloves
- ¼ teaspoon ground cinnamon
- 2 cans (15 ounces each) peach halves in extra-light syrup, drained but retain the juice
- ¼ teaspoon grated orange zest

NUTRITIONAL VALUES PER SERVING: ½ CUP	
Calories	62
Fat	0 g
Carbohydrates	16 g
Protein	0 g
Sodium	7 mg
Potassium	104 mg
Phosphorus	16 mg

DIRECTIONS:

1. Add cornstarch and all the spices into a saucepan. Add retained juice from the cans of the peaches and stir.
2. Place the saucepan over medium heat. Keep stirring until thick. When the mixture starts boiling, lower the heat and cook for 3-4 minutes. Turn off the heat and let it cool until warm. Serve.

256. COCONUT CHOCOLATE ALMOND MOUSSE (VEGAN)

Prep. time: 5 min | Cooking time: 10 min + chilling time | Servings: 8

INGREDIENTS:

- 2 cans (13.5 ounces each) full-fat coconut milk
- 4-6 tablespoons powdered sugar or powdered monk fruit sweetener
- 1 teaspoon vanilla extract
- ½ cup unsweetened cocoa powder
- 4-6 tablespoons unsalted almond butter
- A pinch sea salt

OPTIONAL TOPPINGS:
- Almond slivers
- Whipped coconut milk
- Chocolate shavings
- Raspberries

NUTRITIONAL VALUES PER SERVING: ⅓ CUP (WITHOUT SERVING OPTIONS)	
Calories	218
Fat	20.2 g
Carbohydrates	10.7 g
Protein	4.2 g
Sodium	49.8 mg
Potassium	298 mg
Phosphorus	147.9 mg

DIRECTIONS:

1. Place the coconut milk cans and a mixing bowl along with beaters of the electric hand mixer in the refrigerator for 8-9 hours.
2. Take out the coconut milk cans from the refrigerator carefully so that you do not shake the cans while taking them out.
3. Open the cans and remove the coconut cream that is on the top surface of the coconut milk with a spoon and place it in the chilled bowl.
4. Retain the coconut milk that is remaining in the cans.
5. Fix the beater to the hand mixer and whip the coconut cream until soft peaks are formed. If the peaks are very stiff, you can add 1-2 tablespoons of coconut milk that is remaining in the can and whip until soft peaks are formed.
6. Combine powdered sugar and cocoa in a bowl. Add the cocoa mixture into the mixing bowl and whip until well-incorporated.
7. Beat in the vanilla, almond butter, and salt. Spoon the mixture into 8 small ramekins or glasses.
8. Cover the ramekins with cling wrap and chill for a few hours.
9. Top with optional toppings if desired and serve.

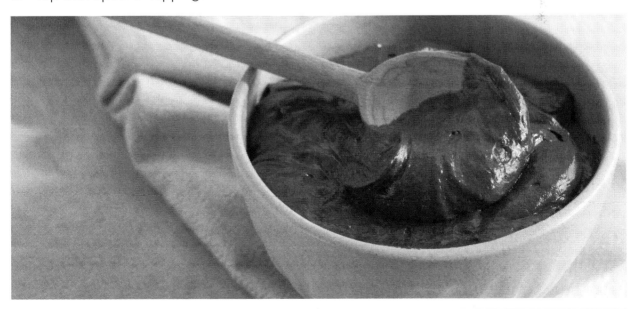

257. POACHED PEARS

Prep. time: 5 min | Cooking time: 30 min | Servings: 2

INGREDIENTS:

NUTRITIONAL VALUES PER SERVING: ½ A PEAR	
Calories	165
Fat	5 g
Carbohydrates	30 g
Protein	0 g
Sodium	31 mg
Potassium	131 mg
Phosphorus	13 mg

- ½ teaspoon ground cinnamon
- 1 Anjou pear, halved, cored (do not peel)
- 1 cup cranberry juice
- 1 teaspoon sugar
- 2 teaspoons butter

DIRECTIONS:

1. Preheat the oven to 350°F. Combine cinnamon and sugar in a bowl.
2. Put the pear halves in a baking dish with the skin side touching the baking dish. In case the pear halves are tumbling off, cut off a thin slice from the rounded part of the pear so that they can stand. Scatter cinnamon sugar on the cut part of the pears. Put a teaspoon of butter in the cavity of the pear (cored part).
3. Drizzle the cranberry juice all around the pear halves. Keep the baking dish covered with foil and place the baking dish in the oven. Bake until fork tender, around 30 minutes.

258. SWEET POPCORN BALLS

Prep. time: 10 min | Cooking time: 10 min | Servings: 9

INGREDIENTS:

NUTRITIONAL VALUES PER SERVING: 1 BALL	
Calories	241
Fat	5 g
Carbohydrates	48 g
Protein	1 g
Sodium	80 mg
Potassium	81 mg
Phosphorus	26 mg

- 8 cups air popped popcorn, unsalted
- 1 cup brown sugar
- ½ tablespoon vinegar
- 1 cup Karo dark corn syrup
- ½ cup water
- 2 tablespoons whipped butter

DIRECTIONS:

1. Combine brown sugar, corn syrup, vinegar, and water in a saucepan. Place the saucepan and keep stirring until it starts boiling.
2. Cook until very thick. Take a drop of the syrup and drop it into a bowl of very chilled water. It should harden instantly. If it doesn't harden, cook for a few more minutes.
3. Turn off the heat. Stir in butter immediately.
4. Place popcorn in a large bowl. Drizzle the syrup over the popcorn. As you drizzle, keep stirring.
5. Make 9 equal sized balls from the mixture.
6. Keep the balls wrapped in cling wrap, wrap each ball separately.
7. Place in an airtight container.

259. APPLE AND BLUEBERRY CRISP

Prep. time: 15 min | Cooking time: 45 min | Servings: 4

INGREDIENTS:

CRISP:
- ½ cup + ⅛ cup quick cooking rolled oats
- 2 tablespoons unbleached all-purpose flour
- 2 tablespoons brown sugar
- 3 tablespoons non-hydrogenated margarine, melted

FILLING:
- ¼ cup brown sugar
- 2 cups fresh or frozen blueberries (do not thaw if frozen)
- ½ tablespoon margarine, melted
- 2 teaspoons cornstarch
- 1 cup grated or chopped apples
- ½ tablespoon lemon juice

NUTRITIONAL VALUES
PER SERVING: ½ CUP COOKED
FRUIT WITH ¼ CUP CRUMBLE

Calories	318
Fat	12 g
Carbohydrates	52 g
Protein	3.3 g
Sodium	148 mg
Potassium	196 mg
Phosphorus	93 mg

DIRECTIONS:

1. Place the rack in the center of the oven. Preheat the oven to 350°F.
2. For crisp: Add oats, flour, and brown sugar into a bowl and mix until well combined. Add margarine and mix until crumbly in texture.
3. To make filling: Add brown sugar and cornstarch into a square baking dish of about 6 inches. Mix well. Add blueberries, margarine, apple, and lemon juice and mix well.
4. Sprinkle the crisp over the filling.
5. Place the baking dish in the oven and set the timer for about 30-45 minutes or until golden brown and crisp on top.
6. Remove from the oven and let it cool for a few minutes before serving. It can be served cold as well.

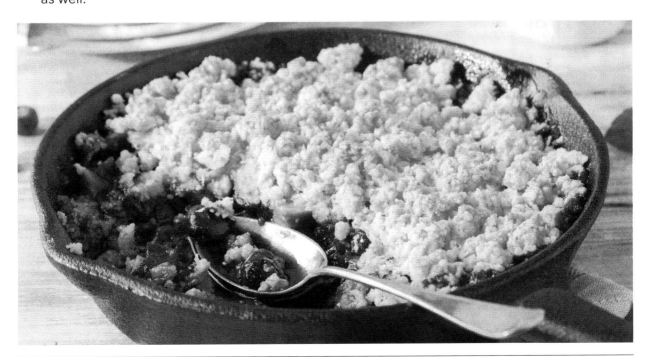

260. SWEET CHERRY COBBLER

Prep. time: 15 min | Cooking time: 15-20 min | Servings: 5

INGREDIENTS:

FILLING:
- 2 ½ cups pitted, halved sweet red cherries
- 1 tablespoon cornstarch
- 1 tablespoon lemon juice
- ⅛ teaspoon almond extract
- ½ teaspoon vanilla extract
- ⅓ cup granulated sugar
- ⅛ teaspoon salt

TOPPING:
- ½ cup all-purpose flour
- ½ teaspoon baking powder
- ⅛ teaspoon ground cinnamon
- ¼ cup nonfat, cold milk
- ¼ cup sugar
- ⅛ teaspoon salt
- 1 tablespoon unsalted, cold butter, cubed

NUTRITIONAL VALUES PER SERVING: ⅙ OF THE RECIPE	
Calories	177
Fat	2 g
Carbohydrates	40 g
Protein	2 g
Sodium	103 mg
Potassium	186 mg
Phosphorus	65 mg

DIRECTIONS:

1. Preheat the oven to 450°F.
2. To make cherry filling: Add cherries, cornstarch, lemon juice, almond extract, vanilla extract, sugar, and salt into a saucepan. Place the saucepan over medium heat. Cook until cherries are cooked and the juices get thick. Turn off the heat.
3. Spoon the filling into a small baking dish. The dish is not to be greased.
4. For topping: Add flour, baking powder, cinnamon, sugar, and salt into a bowl and stir until well combined. Add butter and cut it into the mixture with a fork or pastry cutter until crumbly.
5. Add milk, a little at a time and mix well each time until soft dough is formed. All the milk may not be required. Use as much milk as required. Drop a spoonful of the dough at different spots over the filling. Leave some space between the dough.
6. Place the baking dish in the oven and set the timer for 15-20 minutes, until golden brown on top.
7. Take out the baking dish from the oven and let it cool until warm.
8. Serve. The leftovers, if any, can be refrigerated. Consume within a week but make sure to warm it up before serving.

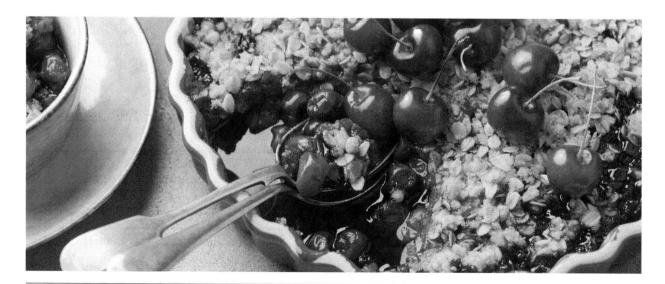

261. FRUIT RUGELACH

Prep. time: 20 min + time for filling | Cooking time: 25-30 min | Servings: 12

INGREDIENTS:

- 1 small egg, separated
- ¼ cup unsalted butter
- 1 cup all-purpose flour
- ¼ teaspoon ground cinnamon
- 6 ounces canned raspberry pie filling
- 2 ½ tablespoons granulated sugar
- 1 teaspoon water
- 2 ounces cream cheese, softened at room temperature

NUTRITIONAL VALUES PER SERVING: 2 FRUIT RUGELACH	
Calories	108
Fat	2 g
Carbohydrates	12 g
Protein	2 g
Sodium	21 mg
Potassium	37 mg
Phosphorus	24 mg

DIRECTIONS:

1. Add flour, cream cheese, 1 ½ tablespoons sugar, butter, and yolk into a mixing bowl and mix well using your hands until dough is formed.
2. Keep the dough wrapped in cling wrap and place it in the refrigerator for 2-8 hours.
3. Preheat the oven to 350°F.
4. Divide the dough into 4 equal portions and shape into balls.
5. Prepare a baking sheet by lining it with parchment paper.
6. Combine remaining sugar and cinnamon in a bowl.
7. Dust your countertop with some flour. Place a ball of dough and roll into a round shape of around ⅛ inch thickness. Place the other balls of dough in the refrigerator until these are made.
8. Spread ¼ of the raspberry pie filling over the dough, leaving the edges. Cut into 6 equal wedges with a pizza cutter.
9. Separate the wedges from each other. Roll each wedge, from the wide side towards the thinner side, finally to the tip of the wedge.
10. Place on the baking sheet, with the seam side facing down.
11. For egg wash: Beat egg white and water in a bowl.
12. Brush the top of the rolls with egg wash. Sprinkle half the cinnamon sugar over the rolls.
13. Repeat the same process with other balls of dough.
14. Place the baking sheet in the oven and bake for about 25-30 minutes or until golden brown on top. Once they are baked, place them on a wire rack and let them cool completely.

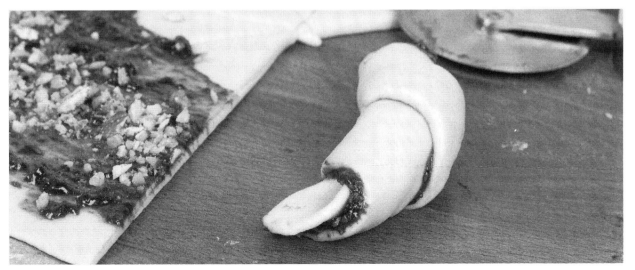

262. SOFT GINGER COOKIES

Prep. time: 20 min | Cooking time: 10 min | Servings: 12

INGREDIENTS:

- 1 ⅛ cups all-purpose flour
- ½ teaspoon baking soda
- ¼ teaspoon ground cloves
- 9 tablespoons sugar
- 2 tablespoons molasses
- 1 teaspoon ground ginger
- 6 tablespoons unsalted butter
- ½ teaspoon ground cinnamon
- 2 tablespoons liquid low-cholesterol egg substitute

NUTRITIONAL VALUES PER SERVING: 1 COOKIE	
Calories	142
Fat	6 g
Carbohydrates	21 g
Protein	2 g
Sodium	60 mg
Potassium	70 mg
Phosphorus	18 mg

DIRECTIONS:

1. Preheat the oven to 450°F.
2. Combine all the dry ingredients in a bowl, i.e. flour, baking soda, and spices.
3. Place butter in a mixing bowl. Set the mixer on medium speed and beat for 30 seconds.
4. Add 8 tablespoons of sugar and beat well.
5. Beat in the molasses and liquid egg substitute. Add flour mixture and mix into dough.
6. Divide the mixture into 9 equal portions and shape into balls. Dredge the balls in a tablespoon of sugar. Place the dough balls on a baking sheet (do not grease the baking sheet). Leave a sufficient gap between the dough balls.
7. Place the baking sheet in the oven and bake for just 10 minutes or until they look light brown, making sure not to bake for as long as you want soft cookies.
8. Let the cookies cool on the baking sheet for a couple of minutes. Now place them on a wire rack to cool completely. Serve.

263. ALMOND MERINGUE COOKIES

Prep. time: 15 min | Cooking time: 25 min | Servings: 12

INGREDIENTS:

- 1 egg white or 2 tablespoons pasteurized egg whites, at room temperature
- ¼ teaspoon vanilla extract
- ¼ teaspoon almond extract
- 3 tablespoons white sugar
- ½ teaspoon cream of tartar

NUTRITIONAL VALUES PER SERVING: 2 COOKIES	
Calories	37.9
Fat	0 g
Carbohydrates	9 g
Protein	0.6 g
Sodium	18 mg
Potassium	51 mg
Phosphorus	0.85 mg

DIRECTIONS:

1. Preheat the oven to 300°F. Prepare a baking sheet by lining it with parchment paper.
2. Add egg white and cream of tartar into a bowl. Beat with an electric hand mixer until frothy and double its original quantity.
3. Add sugar, vanilla, and almond extract and continue beating until you get stiff peaks.
4. Drop 1 teaspoon of the batter on the prepared baking sheet. Use the help of one more teaspoon to drop the batter onto the baking sheet.
5. Place the baking sheet in the oven and set the timer for about 25 minutes or until they turn crisp.
6. Remove from the oven and cool completely.
7. Transfer into an airtight container.

264. FESTIVE COOKIES

Prep. time: 15 min | Cooking time: 7-9 min + chilling time | Servings: 24

INGREDIENTS:

- ½ cup sugar
- 1.5 ounces cream cheese, softened
- ¼ teaspoon salt
- ¼ teaspoon vanilla extract
- ⅛ teaspoon almond extract
- 1 ⅛ cups all-purpose flour
- ½ cup unsalted butter, softened at room temperature
- 1 small egg, separated
- Colored sugar to garnish (optional)

NUTRITIONAL VALUES PER SERVING: 1 COOKIE	
Calories	79
Fat	5 g
Carbohydrates	9 g
Protein	1 g
Sodium	33 mg
Potassium	11 mg
Phosphorus	11 mg

DIRECTIONS:

1. Place sugar, cream cheese, butter, salt, yolk, vanilla, and almond extract in a mixing bowl. Beat with an electric hand mixer until well combined.
2. Place the dough in a bowl. Cover with cling wrap and place it in the refrigerator for about 2 hours.
3. Preheat the oven to 350°F.
4. Dust your countertop with some flour. Place the dough on your countertop and roll the dough into a log with your hand. Cut into 24 equal pieces. Roll the dough balls with a rolling pin until ¼ inch thick.
5. Place the rolled cookies on a baking sheet (do not grease the baking sheet) making sure to leave sufficient gaps between the cookies.
6. Brush with egg white if desired. Scatter colored sugar if using. Place the baking sheet in the oven and bake until light golden brown, around 7-9 minutes.
7. Let the cookies cool completely. Transfer into an airtight container.

265. SNICKERDOODLES

Prep. time: 15 min | Cooking time: 8-10 min | Servings: 12

INGREDIENTS:

- 1 ¼ cups + ⅛ cup all-purpose white flour
- ½ cup butter, softened at room temperature
- 1 teaspoon cream of tartar
- ½ teaspoon vanilla extract
- ¾ cup + ⅛ cup sugar, divided
- 1 egg
- ½ teaspoon baking soda
- ¾ teaspoon ground cinnamon

NUTRITIONAL VALUES PER SERVING: 2 COOKIES	
Calories	185
Fat	9 g
Carbohydrates	24 g
Protein	2 g
Sodium	60 mg
Potassium	66 mg
Phosphorus	26 mg

DIRECTIONS:

1. Preheat the oven to 350°F. Combine flour, cream of tartar, baking soda, and ¾ cup sugar in a bowl.
2. Add butter, vanilla, and egg and mix until dough is formed.
3. Combine ⅛ cup sugar and cinnamon in a shallow bowl.
4. Divide the cookie dough into 24 equal portions and shape into balls.
5. Dredge the dough balls in cinnamon sugar and place on a baking sheet, leaving a sufficient gap between the balls. The baking sheet is not to be greased.
6. Place the baking sheet in the oven and bake for 8-10 minutes or until brown.

266. CREAM CHEESE THUMBPRINT COOKIES

Prep. time: 15 min | Cooking time: 10-12 min + chilling time | Servings: 12

INGREDIENTS:

- ½ cup unsalted butter, softened at room temperature
- 1 cup all-purpose
- 1 teaspoon baking powder
- ¼ cup strawberry jam
- 4 ounces cream cheese
- 1 tablespoon granulated sugar
- ½ teaspoon vanilla extract
- 1 tablespoons powdered sugar

NUTRITIONAL VALUES PER SERVING	
Calories	162
Fat	11 g
Carbohydrates	15 g
Protein	2 g
Sodium	74 mg
Potassium	33 mg
Phosphorus	31 mg

DIRECTIONS:

1. Preheat the oven to 350°F.
2. Combine all the dry ingredients in a bowl, i.e. flour, baking soda, and sugar.
3. Place butter, vanilla, and cream cheese in a mixing bowl. Set the mixer on medium speed and beat until creamy and light.
4. Add flour mixture and mix into dough. Wrap the dough in cling wrap and place it in the refrigerator for 2 hours.
5. Dust your countertop with flour. Place the dough on your countertop and roll the dough using a rolling pin until it is around ¼ inch thick.
6. Using a 1 ½ inch cookie cutter cut out the cookies from the rolled dough.
7. Place the cookies on a baking sheet (do not grease the baking sheet). Leave sufficient gap between the dough balls.
8. You can collect the scrap dough and re-roll the scrap into a small ball of dough. Repeat step 5-7 and cut out some more cookies.
9. Make indentations in the center of each cookie with your thumb. Place ¼ teaspoon jam in the center of each cookie.
10. Place the baking sheet in the oven and bake for 10-12 minutes.
11. Let the cookies cool on the baking sheet for a couple of minutes. Now place them on a wire rack to cool completely.
12. Serve. Store the leftover cookies in an airtight container.

267. ORANGE AND CINNAMON BISCOTTI

Prep. time: 15 min | Cooking time: 60 min | Servings: 9

INGREDIENTS:

- ½ cup sugar
- 1 large egg
- ½ teaspoon vanilla extract
- ½ teaspoon cream of tartar
- ½ teaspoon ground cinnamon
- ¼ cup unsalted butter, at room temperature
- 1 teaspoon grated orange peel
- 1 cup all-purpose flour
- ¼ teaspoon baking soda
- ⅛ teaspoon salt

NUTRITIONAL VALUES PER SERVING: 1 COOKIE	
Calories	149
Fat	6 g
Carbohydrates	22 g
Protein	2 g
Sodium	76 mg
Potassium	53 mg
Phosphorus	28 mg

DIRECTIONS:

1. Preheat The oven to 325°F.
2. Combine all the dry ingredients in a bowl, i.e. flour, cinnamon, salt, baking soda, and cream of tartar. Place butter in a mixing bowl. Set the mixer on medium speed and beat for 30 seconds.
3. Add sugar and beat well. Add egg and beat well. Add orange peel and vanilla and beat until smooth.
4. Add the mixture of dry ingredients into the mixing bowl and mix until well-combined and dough is formed. Chill the dough for 10-15 minutes if possible.
5. Roll the dough into a log of about 4 ½-5 inches long.
6. Place the log on a baking sheet and bake for 35 minutes.
7. Take the baking sheet out of the oven and let the baked log rest for 10 minutes.
8. Cut into 9 slices of ½ inch each. Place them back on the baking sheet with the cut side down. Place the baking sheet back in the oven and bake for 12 minutes. Turn the cookies over and bake for another 12 minutes. Place the baked cookies on a wire rack to cool completely.

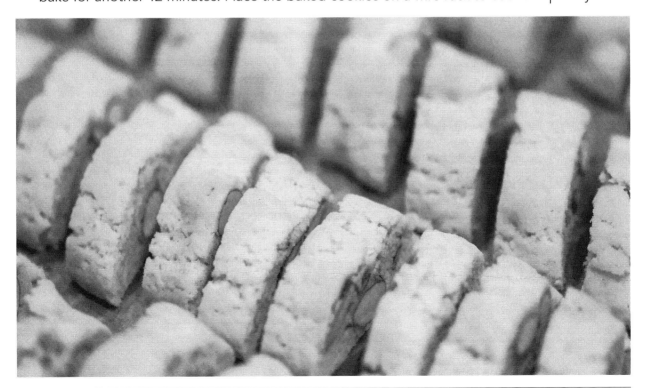

268. PUMPKIN CREAM CHEESE MUFFINS

Prep. time: 20 min | Cooking time: 30 min | Servings: 8

INGREDIENTS:

- 2.7 ounces cream cheese
- 1-1 ½ tablespoons powdered stevia
- ⅔ cup all-purpose flour
- A pinch baking soda
- ⅔ teaspoon baking powder
- 2 tablespoons applesauce
- 6 ½ tablespoons pumpkin puree
- ⅔ teaspoon vanilla extract
- 1 egg
- 9 tablespoons sugar
- ⅓ tablespoon ground cinnamon

NUTRITIONAL VALUES PER SERVING: 1 MUFFIN	
Calories	145
Fat	4 g
Carbohydrates	25 g
Protein	2.5 g
Sodium	78 mg
Potassium	62 mg
Phosphorus	44 mg

DIRECTIONS:

1. Preheat the oven to 375°F. Prepare 8 muffin cups by greasing them with some cooking spray. Place disposable liners in the muffin cups.
2. Beat the egg and add ⅓ of the beaten egg into a bowl. Add cream cheese and stevia and stir until well-combined. Keep it aside.
3. Add remaining egg, pumpkin puree, vanilla, and applesauce into another bowl and whisk well.
4. Combine flour, baking soda, baking powder, cinnamon, and sugar in a 3rd bowl.
5. Add the flour mixture into the bowl of pumpkin puree mixture and stir until just combined, making sure not to over-mix. Divide half the batter among the muffin cups. Divide the cream cheese mixture among the muffin cups.
6. Divide the remaining batter among the muffin cups. Place the muffin cups in the oven and set the timer for 20-25 minutes or until golden brown on top.

269. FUDGE

Prep. time: 5 min | Cooking time: 10-12 min | Servings: 9

INGREDIENTS:

- ⅓ cup half and half creamer
- ¾ cup miniature marshmallows
- ½ teaspoon vanilla extract
- ½ cup + ⅓ cup sugar
- ¾ cup semi-sweet chocolate chips

NUTRITIONAL VALUES PER SERVING: 1 PIECE	
Calories	177
Fat	5 g
Carbohydrates	32 g
Protein	1 g
Sodium	10 mg
Potassium	64 mg
Phosphorus	27 mg

DIRECTIONS:

1. Spray a small square pan (about 5-6 inches) with some cooking spray.
2. Add sugar and half and half into a heavy bottomed pan. When the mixture starts boiling, lower the heat and keep stirring for another 3-4 minutes.
3. Turn off the heat. Stir in chocolate chips, marshmallows, and vanilla. Keep stirring until the marshmallow melts completely.
4. Spoon the mixture into the prepared pan. Let it come to room temperature.
5. Cut into 9 equal pieces and serve. Store the leftover fudge in an airtight container in the refrigerator.

270. CRANBERRIES IN SNOW

Prep. time: 40 min | Cooking time: 10-12 min + chilling time | Servings: 7-8

INGREDIENTS:

- ½ cup cran-cherry juice
- 6 ounces fresh cranberries
- 1 cup granulated sugar
- 4 ounces cream cheese, softened at room temperature.
- 1 packet Knox unflavored gelatin
- ½ cup canned, crushed pineapple in juice, drained
- 1 ½ cups Reddi-Wip dairy whipped topping

NUTRITIONAL VALUES PER SERVING: ½ CUP	
Calories	210
Fat	7 g
Carbohydrates	35 g
Protein	2 g
Sodium	58 mg
Potassium	65 mg
Phosphorus	25 mg

DIRECTIONS:

1. Pour cran-cherry juice into a saucepan. Place the saucepan over medium heat.
2. When it starts boiling, stir in the cranberries. When it starts boiling once again, lower the heat to medium-low heat and simmer until the berries are cooked.
3. Turn off the heat. Add gelatin and 10 tablespoons of sugar and keep stirring until sugar melts. Allow it to cool for about 20 minutes.
4. Add pineapple and stir. Take 7-8 dessert glasses and pour ⅓ cup of the mixture into each glass. Place the glasses in the refrigerator for a couple of hours or until set.
5. Add remaining sugar into a bowl. Add cream cheese and beat with an electric hand mixer until creamy. Add whipped topping and fold in gently. Divide the cream cheese mixture equally and spread over the set cranberry mixture. Chill for an hour or two and serve.

271. BANANA PUDDING DESSERT

Prep. time: 10 min | Cooking time: 10 min + chilling time | Servings: 6

INGREDIENTS:

- 6 ounces vanilla wafers
- 1 box Jell-O cook and serve banana cream pudding mix (3.5 ounces)
- 4 ounces dairy whipped topping
- 1 ¼ cups un-enriched rice milk

NUTRITIONAL VALUES PER SERVING: ⅙ RECIPE	
Calories	259
Fat	7 g
Carbohydrates	46 g
Protein	3 g
Sodium	276 mg
Potassium	52 mg
Phosphorus	40 mg

DIRECTIONS:

1. Take a square or rectangular pan of about 6 inches and spread half the vanilla wafers in it.
2. Combine banana pudding mix and rice milk in a saucepan and place the saucepan over medium heat.
3. Keep stirring until it starts boiling. Turn off the heat. Drizzle the mixture all over the wafers. Place remaining wafers all over the dish and press it gently.
4. Cover the pan and chill for an hour. Spoon the whipped topping over the wafers. Chill for 2-4 hours and serve.

272. BERRIES NAPOLEON BERRIES NAPOLEON

Prep. time: 10 min | Cooking time: 5 min | Servings: 3

INGREDIENTS:

- 6 wonton wrappers
- ¼ cup blueberries
- ¼ cup raspberries
- 1 tablespoon granulated sugar
- Mint leaves to garnish
- ½ tablespoon powdered sugar
- ½ cup Reddi-Wip fat-free whipped topping

NUTRITIONAL VALUES PER SERVING: 1 FILLED WONTON	
Calories	97
Fat	1 g
Carbohydrates	20 g
Protein	2 g
Sodium	100 mg
Potassium	50 mg
Phosphorus	25 mg

DIRECTIONS:

1. Preheat the oven to 400°F. Grease a baking sheet by spraying it with cooking spray.
2. Place the wonton wrappers on the baking sheet without overlapping. Spray the top of the wrappers with cooking spray.
3. Scatter granulated sugar on top of the wrappers.
4. Place the baking sheet in the oven and bake for 5 minutes or until golden brown.
5. Take 6 of the wrappers and place them on a serving platter.
6. Place 2 tablespoons of whipped topping on each wrapper. Place a tablespoon each of blueberries and raspberries on each wrapper.
7. Place a wrapper on each. Scatter powdered sugar on top. Spoon some whipped topping on each, over the wrapper. Top with remaining berries and serve right away.

273. DESSERT CUPS WITH FRESH FRUIT

Prep. time: 10 min | Cooking time: 12 min | Servings: 6

INGREDIENTS:

- 2 phyllo pastry sheets (14 x 18 inches)
- ½ cup fresh blueberries
- ½ cup fresh raspberries
- ½ cup fresh blackberries
- ½ cup fresh strawberries
- Butter flavored nonstick cooking spray
- 1 ½ cups Cool Whip frozen dessert topping

NUTRITIONAL VALUES PER SERVING: 1 DESSERT CUP	
Calories	111
Fat	4 g
Carbohydrates	18 g
Protein	2 g
Sodium	51 mg
Potassium	83 mg
Phosphorus	14 mg

DIRECTIONS:

1. Preheat the oven to 400°F.
2. Grease a 6 count muffin pan with butter flavored cooking spray.
3. Cut each phyllo sheet into 2 halves. Stack them up together. So you will have 4 sheets in the stack.
4. Cut into squares of 3 ½ inches. Place a stack in each muffin cup. Press it into the cup so that it takes the shape of the cup. Bake for 10-12 minutes or until light brown.
5. Take out the muffin pan and let it cool completely. Remove the phyllo cups from the muffin pan.
6. Assemble the cups just before serving. Divide the berries among the cups. Divide the cool whip and place it over berries. Serve.

274. APPLE CINNAMON CUPS

Prep. time: 15 min | Cooking time: 35-40 min | Servings: 3

INGREDIENTS:

FILLING:
- 2 apples, peeled, cored, diced
- 1 tablespoon cold, unsalted butter
- ½ teaspoon ground cinnamon
- 1 tablespoon vanilla extract
- 2 tablespoons light brown sugar
- ⅛ teaspoon ground nutmeg
- ⅛ teaspoon cornstarch

OTHER INGREDIENTS:
- 3 phyllo dough sheets
- 1 tablespoon unsalted butter, melted
- 1 tablespoon ground cinnamon
- 1 ½ tablespoons powdered sugar + extra to garnish if desired
- Mint sprigs to garnish (optional)
- Butter flavored cooking spray

NUTRITIONAL VALUES PER SERVING: 1 CUP	
Calories	280
Fat	13 g
Carbohydrates	38 g
Protein	2 g
Sodium	97 mg
Potassium	177 mg
Phosphorus	33 mg

DIRECTIONS:

1. Preheat the oven to 400°F.
2. Grease 3 large muffin cups with butter flavored cooking spray.
3. To make filling: Add butter into a pan and place the pan over medium heat. When butter melts, add apples and cook for 6-7 minutes until slightly tender.
4. Add cinnamon, brown sugar, and nutmeg and mix well.
5. Stir together vanilla and cornstarch and add into the pan. Keep stirring for a couple of minutes until slightly thick. Remove the pan from heat.
6. Cut each phyllo sheet into 2 halves. Combine powdered sugar and cinnamon in a small bowl. Brush melted butter on either side of a phyllo sheet half and place it on your cutting board.
7. Brush butter on top of the sheet. Sprinkle a little of the cinnamon sugar mixture.
8. Place another phyllo sheet half over this. Repeat the previous step until all the sheet halves, butter, and cinnamon sugar are used up. So you have 6 layers in the stack.
9. Cut into 3 equal pieces. Place a stack in each muffin cup. Press it onto the bottom as well as the sides of the muffin cup as some part will hang out from the edges of the muffin cups.
10. Divide the apple filling equally among the muffin cups. Fold the extra phyllo (that is hanging from the sides of the muffin cups) over the apple filling.
11. Place the muffin cups in the oven and bake for 10-12 minutes or until light golden brown.
12. Take out the muffin cups and let it cool completely.

275. MINI PINEAPPLE UPSIDE DOWN CAKES

Prep. time: 20 min | Cooking time: 40 min | Servings: 24

INGREDIENTS:

- 6 tablespoons unsalted butter, melted
- 24 canned unsweetened pineapple slices
- 1 ⅓ cups sugar
- 6 tablespoons canola oil
- 1 ⅓ cups fat-free milk
- 2 eggs
- 1 teaspoon vanilla extract
- ⅔ cup packed brown sugar
- 12 fresh cherries, halved, pitted
- 2 teaspoons lemon juice
- 2 ⅔ cups cake flour
- ½ teaspoon salt
- 2 ½ teaspoons baking powder

NUTRITIONAL VALUES PER SERVING: 1 CAKE	
Calories	193
Fat	8 g
Carbohydrates	32 g
Protein	3 g
Sodium	131 mg
Potassium	169 mg
Phosphorus	88 mg

DIRECTIONS:

1. Preheat the oven to 400°F.
2. Take 2 muffin pans of 12 counts each and grease it with unsalted melted butter.
3. Scatter a little brown sugar in each muffin cup. Place a slice of pineapple in each muffin cup and press it into the cup so that it takes the shape of the cup.
4. Drop one cherry half in each muffin cup, in the center, with the cut part on top.
5. Add sugar, oil, vanilla extract, milk, and eggs into a bowl and beat until well-incorporated.
6. Mix together flour, salt, and baking powder in another bowl and add it into the bowl of wet ingredients, a little at a time and beat well each time.
7. Divide the batter into the muffin cups in the pan. Place the muffin pans in the oven and set the timer for 35-40 minutes or until cooked through. To check if the cake is done, insert a toothpick in the center of the cake. Remove the toothpick and check if there are any particles stuck on it. If you see any particles stuck on it, you need to bake it for a few more minutes, otherwise turn off the oven and take out the muffin pans. Cool for a few minutes.
8. If necessary, run a knife around the edges of the cake. Invert the cakes onto a plate and serve.

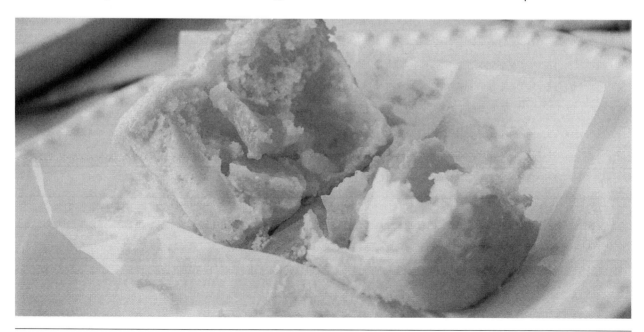

276. APPLE AND CRANBERRY CAKE

Prep. time: 15 min | Cooking time: 60 min | Servings: 24

INGREDIENTS:

- ⅔ cup butter
- 4 eggs
- 3 teaspoons baking soda
- 1 ⅓ cups plain yogurt
- 4 apples, cored, peeled, sliced
- 1 ½ cups sugar
- 3 cups all-purpose flour
- Zest of 2 lemons, grated
- 2 cups cranberries
- 1 cup brown sugar
- 3 teaspoons ground cinnamon

NUTRITIONAL VALUES PER SERVING: 1 SLICE	
Calories	250
Fat	7 g
Carbohydrates	50 g
Protein	3.5 g
Sodium	183 mg
Potassium	110.5 mg
Phosphorus	55 mg

DIRECTIONS:

1. Preheat the oven to 350°F.
2. Prepare a large baking dish of about 10 inches by lining it with parchment paper.
3. Add butter and sugar into a large mixing bowl and beat with an electric hand mixer until creamy.
4. Beat in the eggs, one at a time.
5. Add all the dry ingredients into a bowl, i.e. flour, cinnamon, and baking soda and stir until well-combined.
6. Add dry ingredients into the bowl of butter, a little at a time, along with a little zest and a little yogurt each time. Beat well each time until all the flour mixture, zest, and yogurt is added.
7. Spoon half the batter into the prepared baking dish.
8. Spread cranberries over the batter. Mix together brown sugar and cinnamon in a bowl and sprinkle half of it over the cranberries.
9. Spoon the remaining batter over the cranberries. Spread it evenly.
10. Place the apple slices over the batter. Sprinkle remaining brown sugar mixture over the apples.
11. Place the baking dish in the oven and set the timer for 60 minutes or until golden brown on top. To check if the cake is done, insert a toothpick in the center of the cake. Remove the toothpick and check if there are any particles stuck on it. If you see any particles stuck on it, bake it for a few more minutes, otherwise turn off the oven and take out the baking dish. Cool for a few minutes.
12. Cut into 24 equal slices and serve. Store leftover cake in an airtight container in the refrigerator. Consume within 6-7 days.

277. POUND CAKE

Prep. time: 20 min | Cooking time: 40 min | Servings: 18

INGREDIENTS:

- ½ pound unsalted butter
- 4 large eggs, lightly beaten
- 6 ounces milk
- 1 ½ cups sugar
- 2 ½ cups bread flour
- 1 tablespoon vanilla extract (optional)

NUTRITIONAL VALUES PER SERVING: 1/18 SLICE	
Calories	243
Fat	12 g
Carbohydrates	31 g
Protein	3.7 g
Sodium	18 mg
Potassium	47 mg
Phosphorus	45 mg

DIRECTIONS:

1. Set the temperature ofPreheat
2. Prepare a large baking dish of about 10 inches by lining it with parchment paper.
3. Add butter and sugar into a large mixing bowl and beat with an electric hand mixer until creamy.
4. Beat in the eggs, one at a time. Add vanilla extract if using and beat until well-combined.
5. Add flour and milk and beat until it is well-combined.
6. Pour the batter into the baking dish. Place the baking dish in the oven and bake for about 35-40 minutes or until well-cooked inside.
7. To check if the cake is done, insert a toothpick in the center of the cake. Remove the toothpick and check if there are any particles stuck on it. If you see any particles stuck on it, you need to bake it for a few more minutes, otherwise turn off the oven and take out the baking dish. Cool for about 20 minutes.
8. Cut into 18 equal slices and serve. Store leftover cake in an airtight container in the refrigerator. Consume within 6-7 days.

278. STRAWBERRY PIE

Prep. time: 5 min | Cooking time: 15-20 min + chilling time | Servings: 16

INGREDIENTS:

- 2 pie crusts (9 inches each), unbaked
- 2 cups sugar
- 4 tablespoons lemon juice
- 8 cups chopped strawberries
- 6 tablespoons cornstarch

NUTRITIONAL VALUES PER SERVING: 1 WEDGE	
Calories	246
Fat	8 g
Carbohydrates	44 g
Protein	2 g
Sodium	118 mg
Potassium	146 mg
Phosphorus	30 mg

DIRECTIONS:

1. Follow the instructions given on the package of the pie crusts and bake them.
2. Take them out from the oven and let them cool.
3. Place 4 cups of strawberries in a saucepan and mash them. Add sugar, lemon juice, and cornstarch and place the saucepan over medium heat.
4. Keep stirring until the mixture is thick. Turn off the heat and allow it to cool.
5. Add the remaining strawberries and stir. Divide the mixture among the pie crusts. Cover the crusts with cling wrap and chill for 6-8 hours.
6. Cut each pie into 8 equal wedges and serve.

279. WARM BREAD PUDDING

Prep. time: 10 min | Cooking time: 30 min | Servings: 3

INGREDIENTS:

- 1 egg white
- 1 large egg
- ¾ cup almond milk
- ½ teaspoon vanilla extract
- 1 tablespoon honey
- 1 tablespoon rum or ½ teaspoon rum extract
- 2 slices raisin bread, cut into cubes

NUTRITIONAL VALUES PER SERVING: ½ CUP	
Calories	124
Fat	3 g
Carbohydrates	19 g
Protein	5 g
Sodium	148 mg
Potassium	115 mg
Phosphorus	59 mg

DIRECTIONS:

1. Preheat the oven to 325°F.
2. Grease a small baking dish by spraying it with cooking spray.
3. Add egg and egg white into a bowl and beat until frothy. Add honey, rum, vanilla, and almond milk and whisk until well-combined.
4. Add bread and stir. Spoon the mixture into the baking dish and place it in the oven. Set the timer for 30 minutes or bake until cooked through.
5. To check if the pudding is done, insert a toothpick in the center of the pudding. Remove the toothpick and check if there are any particles stuck on it. If you see any particles stuck on it, bake it for a few more minutes, otherwise turn off the oven and take out the baking dish. Cool for a few minutes. Serve warm.

280. WARM MIXED FRUIT PUDDING

Prep. time: 10 min | Cooking time: 30 min | Servings: 3

INGREDIENTS:

- 2 slices white bread, cut into cubes
- ½ can (from a 15 ounce can) chunky mixed fruit in juice
- ¼ cup unenriched rice milk
- ½ teaspoon ground cinnamon
- 1 ½ tablespoons unsalted butter, melted
- 1 egg

NUTRITIONAL VALUES PER SERVING: ½ CUP	
Calories	210
Fat	9 g
Carbohydrates	31 g
Protein	4 g
Sodium	137 mg
Potassium	185 mg
Phosphorus	66 mg

DIRECTIONS:

1. Preheat the oven to 325°F.
2. Grease a small baking dish by spraying it with cooking spray.
3. Drain the fruits from the can but retain the juice.
4. Combine butter, juice from the can, cinnamon, rice milk, brown sugar, and egg in a bowl. Whisk well. Add fruit and bread cubes and stir until well-incorporated.
5. Spoon the mixture into the baking dish and place it in the oven. Set the timer for 30 minutes or bake until cooked through.
6. To check if the pudding is done, insert a toothpick in the center of the pudding. Remove the toothpick and check if there are any particles stuck on it. If you see any particles stuck on it, bake it for a few more minutes, otherwise turn off the oven and take out the baking dish. Cool for a few minutes. Serve warm.

281. STRAWBERRY PUDDING

Prep. time: 10 min | Cooking time: 5-6 min + chilling time | Servings: 3

INGREDIENTS:

- ½ cup water
- ¼ cup sugar
- 1 cup crushed strawberries
- 1 ¼ tablespoons cornstarch mixed with 2 tablespoons water
- ½ tablespoon fresh lemon juice
- 3 tablespoons whipped dessert topping
- ½ teaspoon grated lemon zest

NUTRITIONAL VALUES PER SERVING: ½ CUP	
Calories	102
Fat	0 g
Carbohydrates	24 g
Protein	0 g
Sodium	2 mg
Potassium	87 mg
Phosphorus	10 mg

DIRECTIONS:

1. Pour water into a saucepan and place the saucepan over medium heat. When it starts boiling, add strawberries and sugar and stir until sugar dissolves.
2. Stir in lemon zest and lemon juice. Keep stirring for a couple of minutes.
3. Add the cornstarch mixture and keep stirring until thick. Turn off the heat.
4. Pour ½ cup mixture into each dessert bowl. Cool completely. Chill for 2-3 hours.
5. Place a tablespoon of whipped topping in each bowl and serve.

282. CRANBERRY FRUIT BARS

Prep. time: 10 min | Cooking time: 40 min | Servings: 12

INGREDIENTS:

CRUST:
- ¾ cup all-purpose flour
- 6 tablespoons unsalted butter, softened at room temperature
- ⅔ cup powdered sugar

FILLING:
- 2 large eggs, beaten
- 4 tablespoons all-purpose flour
- ½ cup dried cranberries
- ½ teaspoon baking powder
- 6 tablespoons sugar
- ½ teaspoon vanilla extract

NUTRITIONAL VALUES PER SERVING: 1 BAR	
Calories	190
Fat	7 g
Carbohydrates	31 g
Protein	2 g
Sodium	34 mg
Potassium	28 mg
Phosphorus	34 mg

DIRECTIONS:

1. To make the crust: Preheat the oven to 350°F.
2. Add flour, butter, and sugar into a bowl. Using your hands, mix until small crumbs are formed.
3. Transfer the mixture into a baking dish of about 8 inches. Press the mixture well.
4. Place the baking dish in the oven and bake for 10-12 minutes until light brown. Take out the baking dish and let it cool for 12-15 minutes.
5. Combine baking powder and flour in a bowl. Add cranberries and toss well.
6. Crack eggs into a bowl. Add vanilla and sugar and beat until well-combined.
7. Stir in the cranberry mixture. Spoon the filling over the crust and place the baking dish back in the oven. Bake for about 20-25 minutes. Take it out of the oven and allow it to cool for about 20 minutes. Slice into 12 equal pieces and serve. You can store the leftover bars in an airtight container in the refrigerator.

283. LEMON BARS

Prep. time: 10 min | Cooking time: 45 min | Servings: 12

INGREDIENTS:

CRUST:
- 1 cup all-purpose flour
- ½ cup unsalted butter, softened at room temperature
- ¼ cup powdered sugar

FILLING:
- ⅛ teaspoon baking soda
- ¾ cup sugar

- ¼ teaspoon cream of tartar
- 2 tablespoons lemon juice
- 2 eggs, beaten
- 2 tablespoons all-purpose flour

GLAZE:
- 1 tablespoon lemon juice
- ½ cup powdered sugar, sifted

NUTRITIONAL VALUES PER SERVING: 1 BAR	
Calories	200
Fat	9 g
Carbohydrates	28 g
Protein	2 g
Sodium	27 mg
Potassium	41 mg
Phosphorus	32 mg

DIRECTIONS:

1. **To make the crust:** Preheat the oven to 325°F.
2. Add flour, butter, and sugar into a bowl. Using your hands, mix until small crumbs are formed.
3. Transfer the mixture into a baking dish of about 8 inches. Press the mixture well.
4. Place the baking dish in the oven and bake for 15-20 minutes, until light brown. Take out the baking dish and let it cool for 12-15 minutes.
5. **To make filling:** Add the dry ingredients into a bowl, i.e. flour, sugar, baking soda, and cream of tartar and mix well
6. Add eggs and lemon juice and whisk until smooth and well-combined.
7. Spoon the filling over the crust and place the baking dish back in the oven. Bake until the top is set. Take it out of the oven and allow it to cool.
8. **Make the glaze:** Combine powdered sugar and lemon juice in a bowl. If the glaze is very thick and you are not able to spread it, add some more lemon juice.
9. Spread the glaze on top. Keep it aside until the glaze sets. Cut into 12 equal sized bars and serve. You can store the leftover bars in an airtight container in the refrigerator.

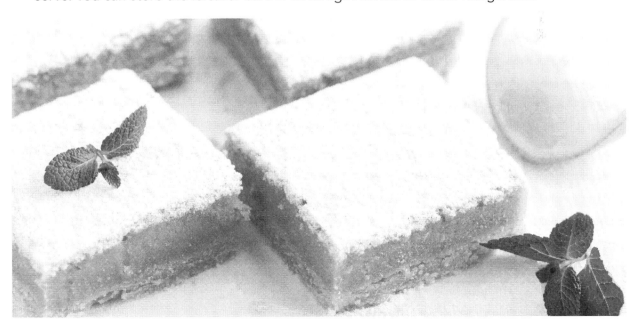

284. PUMPKIN STRUDEL

Prep. time: 20-25 min | Cooking time: 15 min | Servings: 16

INGREDIENTS:

- 3 cups unsalted canned pumpkin
- 2 teaspoons pure vanilla extract
- 1 teaspoon ground cinnamon
- ½ teaspoon grated nutmeg
- 8 tablespoons sugar
- 8 tablespoons unsalted butter, melted
- 24 sheets phyllo dough, thawed if frozen

NUTRITIONAL VALUES PER SERVING: 1 SLICE	
Calories	180
Fat	8 g
Carbohydrates	25 g
Protein	3 g
Sodium	141 mg
Potassium	119 mg
Phosphorus	39 mg

DIRECTIONS:

1. Place the rack in the center of the oven. Preheat the oven to 375°F. Grease a baking sheet with some melted butter.
2. Mix together pumpkin, vanilla, nutmeg, 4 tablespoons sugar, and ½ teaspoon cinnamon in a bowl.
3. Stack 12 phyllo sheets together, brushing in between the sheets lightly with butter. While you are brushing one sheet, make sure the other sheets are covered with a towel or plastic sheet.
4. Make another stack with the remaining 12 phyllo sheets. Make sure to retain some melted butter to brush the top.
5. Divide the pumpkin mixture equally among the stacks and spread it on one edge of the stack.
6. Start rolling from the filling side right up to the opposite edge and place it on the baking sheet with the seam side facing down.
7. Brush remaining butter on top. The top of the rolls should be brushed with butter. Make 3-4 small slits at different spots on the top of each roll.
8. Combine ½ teaspoon cinnamon and 4 tablespoons sugar in a bowl. Scatter this mixture on top of the rolls.
9. Place the baking sheet in the oven and set the timer for about 15 minutes or until golden brown.
10. Once baked, cool for 15 minutes. Cut each roll into 8 equal slices using a sharp knife. Serve.
11. Store leftover strudel in an airtight container in the refrigerator. Warm it up slightly and serve.

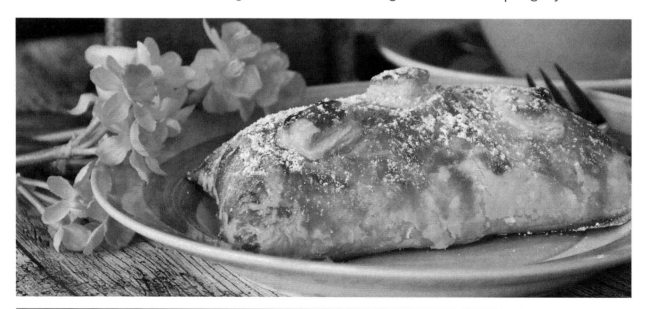

285. CRANBERRY BLONDIES

Prep. time: 20 min | Cooking time: 20 min | Servings: 12

INGREDIENTS:

- 1 ⅛ cups all-purpose flour
- 1 large egg
- ¼ cup dried sweetened cranberries
- 4 ounces cream cheese
- ½ teaspoon ground cinnamon
- 3 tablespoons white chocolate chips
- ¾ cup brown sugar
- ¾ cup powdered sugar
- ½ teaspoon vanilla extract
- ¾ teaspoon baking powder
- 6 tablespoons butter

NUTRITIONAL VALUES PER SERVING	
Calories	217
Fat	10 g
Carbohydrates	29 g
Protein	3 g
Sodium	72 mg
Potassium	53 mg
Phosphorus	44 mg

DIRECTIONS:

1. Place the rack in the center of the oven. Preheat the oven to 350°F. Grease a baking dish with some cooking oil spray or melted butter.
2. Add butter into a saucepan and place it over low heat. When butter melts, turn off the heat.
3. Add brown sugar and stir until it dissolves completely. Pour into a mixing bowl.
4. Once the solution cools completely, add egg and vanilla and beat until well combined.
5. Combine flour and baking powder in a bowl and add into the butter mixture a little at a time and beat well each time.
6. Add white chocolate and about 3 tablespoons of the cranberries and fold in gently.
7. Scoop the batter into the baking dish. Place the baking dish in the oven and set the timer for 20 minutes or bake until cooked through.
8. To check if the Blondies are done, insert a toothpick in the center of the Blondie. Remove the toothpick and check if there are any particles stuck on it. If you see any particles stuck on it, bake it for a few more minutes, otherwise turn off the oven and take out the baking dish. Cool for a few minutes.
9. Cut into 12 equal slices and serve. Store leftover Blondies in an airtight container in the refrigerator. Consume within 6-7 days.

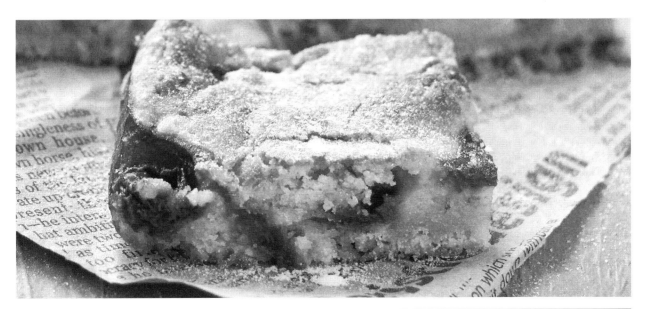

286. APPLE CREPE

Prep. time: 1 hour and 15 min | Cooking time: 40 min | Servings: 4

INGREDIENTS:

- 1 ½ large apples, peeled, cored, sliced
- ½ teaspoon ground cinnamon
- 4 crepes
- 2 tablespoons unsalted butter
- 1 tablespoon brown sugar

- 4 tablespoons whipped topping

CREPE:
- 1 large egg
- ¼ cup all-purpose flour
- ⅔ cup whole milk
- 1 tablespoon butter, melted

NUTRITIONAL VALUES PER SERVING: 1 CREPE WITH ¼ CUP COOKED APPLES AND 1 TBSPABLESPOON WHIPPED TOPPING	
Calories	183
Fat	11 g
Carbohydrates	19 g
Protein	3 g
Sodium	41 mg
Potassium	50 mg
Phosphorus	45 mg

DIRECTIONS:

1. To make batter for crepe: Add egg and milk into a blender and blend until smooth.
2. Add flour and blend once again until you get a smooth batter. Let the batter sit covered in the blender for an hour.
3. Transfer the batter into a bowl. Add butter and whisk well. This quantity of batter will give you 5 crepes. Use 4 in this recipe.
4. Place a nonstick pan or a crepe pan over medium-high heat. Brush some oil or melted butter over it.
5. Take ⅕ of the batter (about ¼ cup) and pour it on the heated pan. Tilt the pan to spread the batter.
6. Cook for about 45 seconds or until the underside is light brown. Turn the crepe over and cook for about 20 seconds.
7. Remove the crepe from the pan and place it on a plate.cCook the remaining crepes similarly.
8. To make filling: While the batter is resting, Preheat the oven to 350°F.
9. Place apples in a baking dish. Drizzle butter over the apples and toss well.
10. Add cinnamon and brown sugar and mix well. Place the baking dish in the oven and bake for 30 minutes or until the apples are cooked.
11. Spread ¼ cup apple mixture on a crepe on the lighter cooked side (the brown side should be down).
12. Roll up the crepes and place on individual serving plates. Place a tablespoon of whipped topping on top and serve.

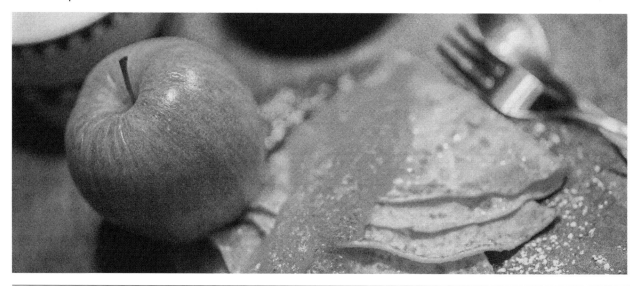

287. BAKED PINEAPPLE

Prep. time: 5 min | Cooking time: 30 min | Servings: 4-5

INGREDIENTS:

- 10 ounces canned crushed pineapple with juice
- A tiny pinch salt
- ¼ teaspoon ground cinnamon
- 1 cup sugar
- 1 large egg, beaten
- 1 ½ tablespoons tapioca
- 1 ½ tablespoons unsalted butter, cold, thinly sliced

NUTRITIONAL VALUES PER SERVING: ½ CUP	
Calories	270
Fat	5 g
Carbohydrates	54 g
Protein	2 g
Sodium	50 mg
Potassium	85 mg
Phosphorus	26 mg

DIRECTIONS:

1. Preheat the oven to 350°F. Combine egg and pineapple in a bowl. Sprinkle salt, tapioca, and sugar over the pineapple and mix well.
2. Transfer the pineapple mixture into a baking dish. Place butter slices over the mixture. Dust with cinnamon and place the baking dish in the oven. Set the timer for 25-30 minutes or until cooked through. This can be served hot or chilled.

288. APPLE FRITTER RINGS

Prep. time: 15 min | Cooking time: 3-4 min per batch | Servings: 10

INGREDIENTS:

- 2 large, tart cooking apples, peeled, cored, cut each into 5 round slices of ½ inch thickness
- 3 tablespoons sugar, divided
- 1 small egg, beaten
- 3 cups almond milk
- 3 tablespoons 1% low-fat milk
- ½ teaspoon canola oil
- ¼ teaspoon ground cinnamon
- ½ cup all-purpose flour
- ½ teaspoon baking powder
- Oil to deep fry, as required

NUTRITIONAL VALUES PER SERVING: 1 FRITTER	
Calories	145
Fat	9 g
Carbohydrates	15 g
Protein	1 g
Sodium	33 mg
Potassium	67 mg
Phosphorus	26 mg

DIRECTIONS:

1. Combine flour, baking powder, and a tablespoon of sugar in a bowl.
2. Whisk together egg, almond milk, milk and oil in another bowl.
3. Pour the milk mixture into the bowl of flour mixture and whisk until just incorporated, making sure not to over-mix.
4. Combine remaining sugar and cinnamon in a small bowl. Keep it aside.
5. Pour enough oil into a small deep frying pan such that the oil is at least 1 inch in height from the bottom of the pan. Let the oil heat to 375°F.
6. Dunk an apple slice in the batter and put it into the hot oil. Place 2-3 apple slices at a time in the hot oil. Cook until they turn golden brown. Turn the apples occasionally.
7. Remove the apples with a slotted spoon and place on a plate lined with paper towels.
8. Cook the remaining apple slices in batches.
9. Sprinkle cinnamon sugar on top of the fritters and serve.

289. ARROZ CON LECHE

Prep. time: 5 min | Cooking time: 20 min | Servings: 3

INGREDIENTS:

- ½ cup uncooked white rice, rinsed
- 1 tablespoon raisins
- 2 tablespoons granulated sugar
- ½ teaspoon vanilla extract
- ½ cup water
- ⅛ teaspoon ground cinnamon
- 1 cup unsweetened almond milk

NUTRITIONAL VALUES PER SERVING: ½ CUP	
Calories	249
Fat	1 g
Carbohydrates	37 g
Protein	3 g
Sodium	60 mg
Potassium	115 mg
Phosphorus	52 mg

DIRECTIONS:

1. Combine rice and water in a small saucepan. Place the saucepan over medium heat. When it starts boiling, lower the heat and cook covered for about 5-6 minutes.
2. Add almond milk and raisins and stir. Continue cooking until the rice is soft. There should be some liquid left in the pot even after the rice is cooked.
3. Turn off the heat. Add sugar, vanilla, and cinnamon. Stir until sugar dissolves completely. Let it cook for 10-15 minutes before serving.

290. FROZEN CRANBERRY DESSERT

Prep. time: 5 min | Cooking time: 5 min + freezing time | Servings: 6

INGREDIENTS:

- 1.5 ounces cherry gelatin mix
- 6 ounces fresh cranberries
- 6 ounces canned jellied cranberry sauce
- 1 cup boiling water
- ¼ cup sugar
- 6 ounces non dairy whipped topping

NUTRITIONAL VALUES PER SERVING: 1 BAR	
Calories	198
Fat	6 g
Carbohydrates	35 g
Protein	1 g
Sodium	35 mg
Potassium	1 mg
Phosphorus	12 mg

DIRECTIONS:

1. Add gelatin mix and ½ cup boiling water in a small bowl.
2. Add sugar and ½ cup boiling into a saucepan Stir until sugar melts. Stir in cranberries and place the saucepan over medium heat. Stir often and bring to a boil. Let it cook for 3-4 minutes. Turn off the heat. Stir in cranberry sauce. Keep whisking until the sauce is chunky.
3. Pour the gelatin mixture and whipped topping and whisk well.
4. Pour into a freezer safe bowl freeze for at least 1-2 hours or until use.

291. BLUEBERRY ICEBOX CAKE

Prep. time: 20 min | Cooking time: 15 min + chilling time | Servings: 5

INGREDIENTS:

- 6 tablespoons unsalted butter
- 3 tablespoons granulated sugar
- 1.5 ounces cream cheese, softened at room temperature
- ¾ cup all-purpose flour
- 1 ½ cups whipped topping
- 10.5 ounces canned blueberry pie filling

NUTRITIONAL VALUES PER SERVING: ⅕ THE RECIPE	
Calories	405
Fat	21 g
Carbohydrates	59 g
Protein	3 g
Sodium	42 mg
Potassium	129 mg
Phosphorus	55 mg

DIRECTIONS:

1. Preheat the oven to 350°F.
2. Combine flour and a tablespoon of sugar in a bowl. Add butter and mix until well-combined and crumbly.
3. Place the mixture in a small square baking dish. Press it well onto the bottom of the dish.
4. Place the baking dish in the oven and set the timer for 15 minutes or until light brown on top. Cool completely.
5. Meanwhile, beat cream cheese with an electric hand mixer until creamy and light.
6. Add remaining sugar and beat until sugar melts.
7. Add whipped topping and fold in gently. Spoon half the cream cheese mixture over the crust. Spread it evenly. Layer with blueberry pie filling followed by remaining cream cheese mixture.
8. Cover the baking dish with cling wrap and place it in the refrigerator for 9-10 hours.
9. Cut into 5 equal slices and serve.

292. RICE CEREAL TREATS

NUTRITIONAL VALUES PER SERVING: 1 BAR	
Calories	77
Fat	1.4 g
Carbohydrates	16 g
Protein	0.5 g
Sodium	11 mg
Potassium	5 mg
Phosphorus	6 mg

Prep. time: 5 min | Cooking time: 10 min | Servings: 3

INGREDIENTS:

- ½ cup mini marshmallows
- 1 ⅓ tablespoons sugar substitute
- 1 cup rice cereal
- 1 teaspoon unsalted butter or margarine

DIRECTIONS:

1. Grease a small, square pan (about 4-5 inches) with some cooking spray or melted butter.
2. Add butter into a small pan and place the pan over low heat. When butter melts, add marshmallows and keep stirring until the marshmallows are melted completely.
3. Stir in sugar substitute. Stir in the rice cereal. Spoon the mixture into the baking dish.
4. Place wax paper over the mixture and press the mixture. On cooling completely, cut into 3 equal slices and serve.

293. FROZEN SUGAR COOKIE SANDWICHES

Prep. time: 20 min | Cooking time: 8-10 min + freezing time | Servings: 8

INGREDIENTS:

- ½ cup unsalted butter, softened at room temperature
- 1 ¼ cups + ⅛ cup all-purpose flour
- ¼ teaspoon baking powder
- 1 small egg
- ¼ cup granulated sugar
- 4 ounces low-fat cream cheese, softened at room temperature
- ½ teaspoon baking soda
- ¾ cup splenda
- 1 teaspoon vanilla extract
- 1 ½ cups Reddi-Wip fat free dairy whipped topping

NUTRITIONAL VALUES PER SERVING: 1 SANDWICH	
Calories	237
Fat	13 g
Carbohydrates	26 g
Protein	4 g
Sodium	142 mg
Potassium	71 mg
Phosphorus	58 mg

DIRECTIONS:

1. Preheat the oven to 375°F.
2. Combine all the dry ingredients in a bowl, i.e. flour, baking powder, and baking soda.
3. Place butter and splenda in a bowl and whisk until smooth. Add egg and ½ teaspoon vanilla extract and beat until well-combined.
4. Add the mixture of dry ingredients and mix until dough is formed. Make 16 equal portions of the mixture and shape into cookies.
5. Place the cookies on a baking sheet (do not grease the baking sheet) and place it in the oven to bake for 8-10 minutes or until light golden brown around the edges.
6. Take out the baking sheet and let the cookies cool completely.
7. Place cream cheese, ½ teaspoon vanilla extract, and sugar in a bowl.
8. Beat with an electric hand mixer until creamy and light.
9. Divide the cream cheese mixture into 8 equal portions. Place one portion in between 2 cookies. Wrap each sandwich separately in foil and freeze until the filling is firm. Serve.

294. RASPBERRY PUNCH

NUTRITIONAL VALUES PER SERVING: ¾ CUP	
Calories	70
Fat	0 g
Carbohydrates	16 g
Protein	1 g
Sodium	8 mg
Potassium	91 mg
Phosphorus	6 mg

Prep. time: 5 min | Cooking time: 0 min | Servings: 12

INGREDIENTS:

- 4 cups diet ginger ale, chilled
- 23 ounces canned pineapple juice
- 8 ounces raspberry sherbet or sorbet
- 5 ounces frozen raspberries, thawed
- 3 ounces frozen pink lemonade concentrate

DIRECTIONS:

Add pineapple juice, sherbet, lemonade, and diet ginger ale into a punch bowl and stir until well-combined. Add raspberries and stir. Serve.

295. COLORFUL PIE

Prep. time: 15 min | Cooking time: 0 min + chilling time | Servings: 16

INGREDIENTS:

- 16 ounces whipped low-fat cream cheese
- 6 cups Reddi-Wip dairy whipped topping
- 2 cups fresh blueberries
- 1 cup low-sugar red raspberry preserves
- 2 prepared graham cracker crusts (9 inches each)
- 3 cups fresh raspberries

NUTRITIONAL VALUES PER SERVING: 1 WEDGE	
Calories	237
Fat	9 g
Carbohydrates	35 g
Protein	4 g
Sodium	220 mg
Potassium	162 mg
Phosphorus	91 mg

DIRECTIONS:

1. For filling: place cream cheese and raspberry preserves in a bowl. Set the electric hand mixer on medium speed and beat until smooth.
2. Add most of the whipped topping and fold gently. Divide the filling equally among the crusts and spread it over the crusts. Place the crusts in the freezer for 30-60 minutes.
3. To decorate: Divide the berries among the crusts. Place the blueberries all around the outer circumference of the pies.
4. Place the raspberries near the blueberries to form the inner circumference.
5. Place some whipped topping in the center of each pie. If there are any raspberries remaining, place them in the center of the pies, over the whipped topping.
6. Cut each pie into 8 equal wedges and serve.

296. RUM PEAR TARTS

Prep. time: 30 min | Cooking time: 5-10 min + chilling time | Servings: 24

INGREDIENTS:

- 1 package vanilla pudding mix (3 ounces)
- 3 teaspoons rum extract
- 2 cups rice milk, un-enriched
- 2 packages (12 counts each) mini phyllo cups
- 2 pears, peeled, cored, cut each into 12 equal pieces

NUTRITIONAL VALUES PER SERVING: 1 TART	
Calories	137
Fat	1.4 g
Carbohydrates	29 g
Protein	1.4 g
Sodium	256 mg
Potassium	79 mg
Phosphorus	118 mg

DIRECTIONS:

1. Follow the directions on the package of the pudding mix and prepare the pudding using rice milk.
2. Stir in rum extract and place it in the refrigerator until very chilled.
3. Divide the pudding among the phyllo cups. You should be able to place 1 heaping teaspoon in each cup. Top with a piece of pear. Serve.

297. SWEET POTATO PIE

Prep. time: 15 min | Cooking time: 1 hour and 20 min | Servings: 16

INGREDIENTS:

- 4 medium sweet potatoes, peeled, cut into cubes
- 1 cup granulated sugar
- 1 ½ cups 2% reduced-fat evaporated milk
- 2 teaspoons ground cinnamon
- 2 unbaked deep dish pastry shell (9 inches)
- ⅔ cup butter
- 4 large eggs, at room temperature
- 2 teaspoons vanilla extract
- 2 teaspoon ground nutmeg

NUTRITIONAL VALUES PER SERVING: 1 WEDGE	
Calories	320
Fat	17 g
Carbohydrates	37 g
Protein	5 g
Sodium	152 mg
Potassium	195 mg
Phosphorus	107 mg

DIRECTIONS:

1. Preheat the oven to 425°F.
2. Boil sweet potatoes in a pot of water until fork tender. Drain the sweet potatoes and add it back into the pot. Mash the sweet potatoes using a potato masher until smooth. Let it cool completely.
3. Place butter and sugar in a mixing bowl. Beat with an electric hand mixer until smooth.
4. Beat in the eggs. Pour milk and vanilla. Add spices and beat until well-combined.
5. Measure out 4 cups of the sweet potatoes and add them into the bowl. Beat until smooth.
6. Divide the mixture into the pie shells. Spread the mixture evenly. Keep the crusts covered with aluminum foil and place them in the oven.
7. After 15 minutes, decrease the temperature of the oven to 350°F and continue baking for about 35-40 minutes. Insert a knife in the center of the filling and take it out. If the knife is clean and has no particles stuck on it, the pies are ready. Let it cool completely.
8. Chill until use. Cut each pie into 8 equal wedges and serve.

298. APPLE CRUMBLE

Prep. time: 15 min | Cooking time: 45 min | Servings: 6

INGREDIENTS:

- 2 large apples, peeled, cored cut into ½ inch thick slices
- ¼ teaspoon ground cinnamon
- ⅛ cup unsalted butter
- ¼ cup oats
- ⅛ cup all-purpose flour
- ¼ cup packed brown sugar
- A tiny pinch salt

NUTRITIONAL VALUES PER SERVING	
Calories	126
Fat	4 g
Carbohydrates	10 g
Protein	17 g
Sodium	17 mg
Potassium	94 mg
Phosphorus	26 mg

DIRECTIONS:

1. Preheat the oven to 350°F.
2. Spread the apple slices in a small baking dish.
3. Mix together oats, flour, brown sugar, salt, and cinnamon in a bowl. Add butter and cut it into the mixture using a pastry cutter.
4. Once the butter is well-combined with the mixture, scatter over the apples.
5. Place the baking dish in the oven and bake until the top side becomes golden brown.

299. BLUEBERRY PEACH CRISP

Prep. time: 10 min | Cooking time: 45-60 min | Servings: 20

INGREDIENTS:

- 2 cups blueberries
- 14 medium peaches, pitted, cut into ¾ inch slices
- ½ cup granulated sugar
- 1 ½ cups all-purpose flour
- 1 cup butter
- 2 tablespoons lemon juice
- 1 ½ cups packed brown sugar

NUTRITIONAL VALUES PER SERVING	
Calories	228
Fat	10 g
Carbohydrates	35 g
Protein	2 g
Sodium	76 mg
Potassium	240 mg
Phosphorus	30 mg

DIRECTIONS:

1. Preheat the oven to 375°F.
2. Grease a large baking dish (13 x 9 inches) with cooking spray.
3. Place peach slices all over the baking dish. Scatter blueberries over the peaches.
4. Scatter granulated sugar all over the fruits. Drizzle lemon juice all over.
5. Combine brown sugar and flour in a bowl. Add butter and cut it into the mixture until you get crumbles. Scatter the crumbles on top.
6. Place the baking dish in the oven and set the timer for 45 minutes or until golden brown on top.
7. Take the dish out of the oven and let it cool until warm. Serve.

300. SHERBET SHAKE

Prep. time: 5 min | Cooking time: 0 min | Servings: 1

INGREDIENTS:

- ¼ cup low-cholesterol egg product
- 1 tablespoon almond milk
- ½ cup sherbet, any flavor

NUTRITIONAL VALUES PER SERVING: ¾ CUP	
Calories	138
Fat	2 g
Carbohydrates	24 g
Protein	6 g
Sodium	133 mg
Potassium	154 mg
Phosphorus	38 mg

DIRECTIONS:

1. Blend together egg product, almond milk, and sherbet in a blender until smooth.
2. Serve right away.

COOKING CONVERSION

WEIGHT COVERSION	
½ oz.	15g
1 oz.	30g
2 oz.	60g
3 oz.	85g
4 oz.	110g
5 oz.	140g
6 oz.	170g
7 oz.	200g
8 oz.	225g
9 oz.	255g
10 oz.	280g
11 oz.	310g
12 oz.	340g
13 oz.	370g
14 oz.	400g
15 oz.	425g
1 lb.	450g

LIQUID VOLUME MEASUREMENTS

TABLESPOONS	TEASPOONS	FLUID OUNCES	CUPS
16	48	8 fl. Oz.	1
12	36	6 fl. Oz.	¾
8	24	4 fl. Oz.	½
5 ½	16	2 ⅔ fl. Oz.	⅓
4	12	2 fl. Oz.	¼
1	3	0.5 fl. Oz.	1/16

LIQUID VOLUME CONVERSION

CUPS / TABLESPOONS	FL. OUNCES	MILLILITERS
1 cup	8 fl. Oz.	240 ml
¾ cup	6 fl. Oz.	180 ml
⅔ cup	5 fl. Oz.	150 ml
½ cup	4 fl. Oz.	120 ml
⅓ cup	2 ½ fl. Oz.	75 ml
¼ cup	2 fl. Oz.	60 ml
⅛ cup	1 fl. Oz.	30 ml
1 tablespoon	½ fl. Oz.	15 ml

TEASPOON (tsp.) / TABLESPOON (Tbsp.)	MILLILITERS
1 tsp.	5ml
2 tsp.	10ml
1 Tbsp.	15ml
2 Tbsp.	30ml
3 Tbsp.	45ml
4 Tbsp.	60ml
5 Tbsp.	75ml
6 Tbsp.	90ml
7 Tbsp.	105ml

TEMPERATURE CONVERSIONS	
CELSIUS	**FAHRENHEIT**
54.5°C	130°F
60.0°C	140°F
65.5°C	150°F
71.1°C	160°F
76.6°C	170°F
82.2°C	180°F
87.8°C	190°F
93.3°C	200°F
100°C	212°F
110°C	220°F
120°C	248°F
130°C	266°F
140°C	284°F
150°C	302°F
160°C	320°F
170°C	338°F
180°C	356°F
190°C	374°F
200°C	392°F
210°C	410°F
220°C	428°F
230°C	446°F
240°C	464°F
250°C	482°F

Conclusion

I want to thank you once again for choosing this book. I hope it proved to be an enjoyable and informative read! Following the renal diet means sticking to a diet that slows down the progression of a renal disorder, promotes recovery, and does not tax your kidneys. Limiting your sodium and potassium intake while increasing the consumption of high-quality protein are important features of a typical renal diet. Do not think of this diet as restrictive. Instead, concentrate on all the ingredients you can consume.

The renal diet is not difficult to follow. All that it requires is some consistent effort and dedication, and you will notice a positive change in your overall health and well-being. After all, taking care of your health is your responsibility and this cannot be outsourced. Living with kidney disease is certainly not easy. That said, this should not prevent you from leading the life you desire. To lead a happy and fulfilling life, taking care of your physical health is essential. This is where the renal diet steps into the picture. This diet is designed keeping in mind the goal of improving the functioning and overall health of your kidneys.

Also, all the information you need to start following this diet is given in this book. From learning about what the diet means to all that it entails and a variety of recipes, this book will act as your guide every step of the way.

Who says following a diet means eating bland and boring meals? Who says you cannot consume delicious meals specifically designed for improving your kidney health? Well, this is what the renal diet is all about. In this book, you were introduced to a variety of renal diet-friendly meals that will help improve your health without compromising on flavors. These recipes focus on natural flavors and wholesome ingredients instead of processed foods that you do not need.

So, what are you waiting for? There is no time like the present to commit to a healthy diet for improving your overall health and well-being. Taking charge of your renal health is within your reach. All you need to do is make a conscious dietary change, stay away from foods that harm kidney health, and focus on increasing the consumption of foods that are good for optimizing kidney functioning. Following this diet is incredibly simple. All that requires is a little patience, commitment, consistency, and dedication. Once you do this, you can improve kidney health and recovery. All the information you need to follow this diet is given in this book.

Now, all that you need to do is clear out your pantry and restock it with the required ingredients. After this, select a recipe that strikes your fancy and follow the simple instructions given in this book. Yes, it is as simple as that! By consistently following the renal diet, you will see a positive change in your kidney health.

Thank you and all the best!

References

8 Golden Rules - World Kidney Day. (2014). World Kidney Day. https://www.worldkidneyday.org/facts/take-care-of-your-kidneys/8-golden-rules/

Betz, M. (2021, May 6). Downloadable Renal Diet Grocery List. The Kidney Dietitian. https://www.thekidneydietitian.org/renal-diet-grocery-list/

Biggers, A. (2019, October 3). 11 Tips to Prevent Kidney Failure, Treatment Options & More. Healthline. https://www.healthline.com/health/kidney-health/how-to-prevent-kidney-failure#11-tips

Borrelli, S., Provenzano, M., Gagliardi, I., Michael, A., Liberti, M. E., De Nicola, L., Conte, G., Garofalo, C., & Andreucci, M. (2020). Sodium Intake and Chronic Kidney Disease. International journal of molecular sciences, 21(13), 4744. https://doi.org/10.3390/ijms21134744

Chronic kidney disease: Exercise provides clear benefits. (2014). ScienceDaily. https://www.sciencedaily.com/releases/2014/11/141115083118.htm

Fang, X., Wei, J., He, X., An, P., Wang, H., Jiang, L., Shao, D., Liang, H., Li, Y., Wang, F., & Min, J. (2015). Landscape of dietary factors associated with risk of gastric cancer: A systematic review and dose-response meta-analysis of prospective cohort studies. European Journal of Cancer, 51(18), 2820–2832. https://doi.org/10.1016/j.ejca.2015.09.010

Goodman, E. (2021, March 24). Low sodium diet: What it is, benefits, foods, and more. Www.medicalnewstoday.com. https://www.medicalnewstoday.com/articles/low-sodium-diet#conditions-it-might-benefit

Helmy, A. Z. (2020, November 25). Low-Sodium Diet: Pros, Cons, And More. LipoSci Labs. https://phenterpro.com/blogs/news/low-sodium-diet-pros-cons-and-more

How Salt Can Impact Your Blood Pressure, Heart and Kidneys. (2017, June 15). Health Essentials from Cleveland Clinic; Health Essentials from Cleveland Clinic. https://health.clevelandclinic.org/kidneys-salt-and-blood-pressure-you-need-a-delicate-balance/

Is too much phosphorus in food a threat to your kidneys? I Center for Science in the Public Interest. (2016). Cspinet.org. https://cspinet.org/tip/too-much-phosphorus-food-threat-your-kidneys

Johnson, I. T. (2015). Understanding the association between diet and nutrition in upper gastrointestinal cancer. Expert Review of Gastroenterology & Hepatology, 9(11), 1347–1349. https://doi.org/10.1586/17474124.2015.1088383

Ko, G. J., Obi, Y., Tortorici, A. R., & Kalantar-Zadeh, K. (2017). Dietary protein intake and chronic kidney disease. Current Opinion in Clinical Nutrition and Metabolic Care, 20(1), 77–85. https://doi.org/10.1097/mco.0000000000000342

Let's Get Active! Exercise for Kidney Patients. (n.d.). National Kidney Federation. https://www.kidney.org.uk/lets-get-active-exercise-for-kidney-patients

Managing Chronic Kidney Disease | NIDDK. (2019, September 19). National Institute of Diabetes and Digestive and Kidney Diseases. https://www.niddk.nih.gov/health-information/kidney-disease/chronic-kidney-disease-ckd/managing

Picard, K., Barreto Silva, M. I., Mager, D., & Richard, C. (2020). Dietary Potassium Intake and Risk of Chronic Kidney Disease Progression in Predialysis Patients with Chronic Kidney Disease: A Systematic Review. Advances in Nutrition, 11(4), 1002–1015. https://doi.org/10.1093/advances/nmaa027

Rubio-Aliaga, I. (2020). Phosphate and Kidney Healthy Aging. Kidney and Blood Pressure Research, 45(6), 802–811. https://doi.org/10.1159/000509831

Wang, M., Moran, A. E., Liu, J., Qi, Y., Xie, W., Tzong, K., & Zhao, D. (2015). A Meta-Analysis of Effect of Dietary Salt Restriction on Blood Pressure in Chinese Adults. Global Heart, 10(4), 291-299. e6. https://doi.org/10.1016/j.gheart.2014.10.009

Made in the USA
Las Vegas, NV
01 December 2022

60710151R00120